Wider Horizons

Care of the Dying in a Multicultural Society

Shirley Firth

July 2001

**National Council
for Hospice
and Specialist
Palliative Care
Services**

© Shirley Firth 2001
ISBN: 1 898915 27 X

Published by the National Council for
Hospice and Specialist Palliative Care Services
1st Floor, 34-44 Britannia Street,
London WC1X 9JG

Tel: 020 7520 8299
Fax: 020 7520 8298
email: enquiries@hospice-spc-council.org.uk
Website: www.hospice-spc-council.org.uk

A company limited by guarantee no. 2644430
Registered as a Charity no. 1005671

Acknowledgements

My thanks to Rasaratnam Balarajan, Roger Ballard, Simon Dein, Elizabeth Anionwu, David Oliviere, Anne Eve, Peter Tebbit, Jonathan Koffman, Anthony Smith, Kelvin Karim, Lalitha Webb, Mercy Jeyasingham, Jennifer Layburn, Mary Haworth, Jan Fish, Alison Shaw, Chris Smaje, Katy Gardner and Yasmin Gunaratnam for discussing various points with me. Peter Aspinall has been unfailingly helpful over census data and ethnic categories. Katy Gardner, Yasmin Gunaratnam, Jaqueline Somerville and Jonathan Koffman kindly allowed me to read their articles prior to publication. My particular thanks go to David Field for editing the document with care and patience. Bee Wee and Sam Ahmedzai read and commented on the script and made many helpful suggestions. Any mistakes are entirely my responsibility. My thanks are also due to Richard Hillier, Bee Wee and Ruth Andrews at Countess Mountbatten Hospice for their assistance in setting up the literature review. Eve Richardson, John Mount and Rosemary Simmonds have given help and encouragement, as have Jayne Thomas and Philippa Casbon at the National Council. My husband, David, and daughter, Katharine, proof read and made useful suggestions, as well as putting up with my preoccupations.

Contents

Introduction

When *Opening Doors* was written in 1995, it was evident that black and ethnic minority people were not utilising hospice and palliative care services in proportion to their numbers. The report claimed that access was limited because of low referral rates, lack of knowledge and information about services, and because black and ethnic minorities preferred to care for dying patients at home. Low rates of cancer were seen as one reason for low uptake, but the figures were likely to have been inaccurate because of poor ethnic monitoring. When the services were utilised there were reported problems of communication and misunderstandings over cultural, religious and gender issues. At the same time there were examples of imaginative attempts to provide a culturally sensitive service.

The study was written from the perspective of care services in two London Health Authorities and one in Birmingham. Service users were not interviewed for the project, and it did not address the different needs of different black and ethnic minority groups, or recognise the differences existing between different groups.

It is evident that despite many excellent research projects and initiatives, many of the issues raised by Hill and Penso in 1995 are still major concerns in ensuring access to, and providing culturally sensitive care for ethnic minority patients.[1] The numbers of ethnic minority patients accessing hospice and palliative care services are still not commensurate with the size of the ethnic minority populations. While cancer rates for most ethnic minority groups are lower than mainstream white populations, these are rising with the ageing of the ethnic minority population and the changes in health due to adaptation to British diet and environment. Those diseases with the highest mortality rates for ethnic minority groups, coronary heart disease (CHD) and hypertension are not

---

1 The term 'ethnic minority' is being used in preference to the commonly used 'Black and ethnic minority' to avoid the racial and political overtones of the latter term. The term 'white' is equally fraught with difficulties, but it is not possible here to explore this issue further, except to point out that the 'white' community is no more homogeneous than the 'black and ethnic minority' communities. (See Bhopal and Donaldson, 1998 and Ch.2 below, fn. 7).

normally cared for within PC services, which raises questions as to whether PC should broaden its remit to include conditions other than cancer. This is being vigorously debated.

Despite the statutory requirement for hospitals to record ethnic data, inadequate ethnic monitoring still makes it difficult to assess accurately either the need for or the use of Hospice and Specialist Palliative Care Services. The bulk of the studies refer to people from the Indian subcontinent and the Caribbean, but there are little or no data on Chinese, Arabs, Turks, Greeks and new immigrants. The few available ethnographic studies make it clear that the needs of patients and carers in specific Bangladeshi and African Caribbean groups are still not being met. Insensitivity, racism and lack of cultural awareness are still evident in the health services generally, including reports of racism, stereotypical thinking, ignorance and confusion on the part of professionals. Racist patients have also challenged staff on the wards. Palliative Care Service provision is based on existing Western models of care.

Current studies on GP services present a mixed picture of good and poor responses to ethnic minority needs. Criticisms are still being made about low rates of referrals of patients with cancer, particularly by GPs, both from the minority and majority communities. Studies of user satisfaction indicate that many patients feel they do not have enough time during GP consultations. Communication is still a major issue for first generation ethnic minority patients, and language problems are seen as a barrier to access to health services. There have been a number of initiatives to improve advocacy, linkworker and interpreter schemes but even where there are interpreting services they are underused or inadequate and reliance on relatives continues despite evidence that this is often inappropriate.

The terminology in use with respect to ethnic minorities is often problematic. Expressions such as 'black and ethnic minority' may be useful in a political context but are also in danger of creating a sense of 'otherness' or difference. This can lead to stereotyping and generalisations. It is important to recognise the heterogeneous nature of all ethnic communities (including 'white' ones) and be aware of the context in which they live, whether in nuclear or extended families, and in situations of dispersal and fragmentation. Varieties of health beliefs, religious and spiritual needs, and ways of coping with emotional and spiritual pain need to be recognised and understood. Ethnically sensitive care has to recognise individual patients' and carers' own worldview and location in the context of the wider community. In particular, the great importance of religion to many ethnic minority people is not sufficiently acknowledged in much of the literature. There appears to be a strong preference for home deaths, which has implications for palliative care. Strong religious and cultural feelings about caring for relatives at home may conflict with a sense of failure and fear of stigma if help is needed with home care, or if it proves impossible.

The roles of professionals such as advocates, linkworkers, doctors and nurses, are discussed. The concepts of cultural competence and cultural safety are relevant to the philosophy and practice of culturally sensitive nursing, both at undergraduate and postgraduate levels. While there appear to be commensurate numbers of ethnic minority and white nurses for the population, there are fewer, proportionately, South Asian nurses, and not enough ethnic minority nurses in palliative care, so there are recruitment issues.

Finally, there is the question of outreach, which involves the provision of adequate information, meeting the communities in various ways through local organisations, and involvement in decision making and management.

Lest this all seems to be gloomy, there are also excellent studies and ongoing fieldwork, taking up some of the issues raised by Hill and Penso, as well as encouraging reports of good practice. For example, the Warwickshire Health Authority Project is specifically addressing the palliative care needs of black and ethnic minority patients in the area (Webb and Young 2000). Studies on Bangladeshi carers (Spruyt 1999 and Somerville 2001) and Black Caribbean Carers (Koffman and Higginson 2001) also provide information about patient needs. There is a comparative study in progress in Leeds, Bradford and Leicester on South Asian needs in palliative care (Ahmad *et al,*)[2]. Sharing information and experiences of good practice will help palliative care services throughout the country to develop their own models further.

The following discussion gives an overview of *Opening Doors*, and then, rather than following the issues raised point by point, reviews literature since 1995,[3] discussing selected issues. These are, broadly speaking, issues of terminology, classification and ethnic monitoring; care for black and ethnic

---

2 This is a qualitative 26-month study entitled 'South Asian and white patients with advanced cancer: patients' and families' experience of the illness and perceived needs for care' jointly funded by the CRC and DoH as part of an initiative on Black and Ethnic Minority Groups and Cancer from 1998. Other contributors to the study are Mary Haworth, Sangeeta Chattoo, Mari Lloyd-Williams and Rosemary Lennard.

3 Where earlier studies are important and relevant to the discussion, they will also be cited.

minorities, including the suitability and appropriate location of specialist palliative care services; religious and spiritual care, the roles and training of professionals (doctors, nurses and advocates/linkworkers); recruitment of ethnic minority staff and outreach. Very little literature was found on community care, on social services provision for ethnic minority patients and families with respect to palliative care, or on discharge and care in nursing and residential homes. This reflects the findings of Hill and Penso, and is thus a gap, which still needs to be addressed. Issues of purchase and provision are also not addressed, as these can be more appropriately dealt with elsewhere. The principle behind this document is to examine ways of improving services from the perspective of black and ethnic minorities themselves, not just to explore questions of uptake.

A summary of key recommendations is included at the end of the document, and it is hoped that this review paves the way for more comprehensive research into the question of ethnic minority access to equitable hospice and specialist palliative care services, and in particular into the gaps which have been identified.

Chapter 1

Overview of *Opening Doors*

1. 1. The objectives in *Opening Doors* were:

- To identify the extent of, and the reasons for, low uptake of hospice and specialist palliative care services.
- To ensure that purchasers and providers were aware of ways in which access and uptake can be improved.
- To develop checklists and guidelines to help providers and to develop services sensitive to black and ethnic minority patients, their families and carers.
- To help purchasers measure ways in which services meet the needs of all the local population.

1.2. Methods

Hill and Penso focused on hospices and palliative care in the hospitals and community in three areas with large ethnic minority populations: Brent in Outer London, Newham in Inner London, and Birmingham. Information was gathered through interviews with professional staff, and from some GPs, although the response of the latter to the questionnaires was disappointing. Patients and carers were not interviewed except for one Asian volunteer. There were uneven gaps in the information provided which may reflect on the questions asked. For example only one institution discussed discharge arrangements, and in only one were there specific references to psychological and social issues, reduced to matters of assistance with welfare, benefits, immediate practical needs and financial matters.

1.3. Findings from *Opening Doors*

1.3.1. Data on ethnic minorities

- There was a lack of accurate data on ethnicity.
- Ethnic monitoring was patchy or non-existent, and the correct recording of names in hospitals was poor.
- There was a lower incidence of cancer among ethnic minorities.
- Service use will increase with ageing.

1.3.2. Access

- Fear of and stigma associated with cancer may prevent ethnic minority patients accessing services.
- There were assumptions that ethnic minorities 'care for their own'.
- Patients from Bangladesh and Pakistan may wish to return to their country of origin to die.
- Hospices may be seen as Christian or inappropriate for Asian patients.
- Appropriate food provision was inadequate.
- Ethnic minority patients were unaware of their entitlements and available services.
- Hospice and specialist palliative care services were sometimes refused.
- Staff attitudes were seen as a reason for low referral rates.
- Low referral rates from both GPs and hospitals.

1.3.3. Cultural issues in care

- Gender issues in care, relating particularly to the way women were treated and cared for.
- Too many relatives around a death bed.
- Disclosure issues associated with beliefs about death and family structures.
- Attempts to meet religious and cultural requirements, but difficulties in understanding some of these.
- Conflicts with western medicine, cultural attitudes and religious beliefs.
- Pain control issues occurred on religious grounds.
- Bereavement support groups were needed.
- Difficulties occurred with discharging patients.
- Facilities for ethnic minority patients were often inadequate (showers, privacy, adequate food, etc.

1.3.4. Religious and spiritual care

- Different attitudes to pain relief.
- Wanting to be conscious at death.
- Needing space for rituals.

1.3.5. Doctors

- There were no patterns of consistent referrals.
- Religious and caste differences between some Asian doctors and patients could be problematical.
- There were few ethnic minority doctors and nurses in hospice and specialist palliative care services.
- Asian GPs were uninformed about hospice and palliative care services.

1.3.6. Service provision

- Ethnic monitoring was patchy; and needed to be linked to referrals.
- Staff training and education needed to be improved.
- There was a need for culturally sensitive services.
- There was a lack of appropriate, accessible information, both for patients (in their appropriate languages) and for staff.
- Health sector organisations and hospices had insufficient data for providing appropriate information.
- Language and communication were often a problem, the use of family members problematic, and interpreting services were generally inadequate, *ad hoc* and used ineffectively.

1.4. Recommendations by Hill and Penso

The report recommended that service delivery had "better overall collaboration between the purchasers and providers in the statutory and voluntary sector" (p.44), within which the role of hospices should be defined. However, the level of training and service provision was seen as dependent on the local population of ethnic minorities, within an Equal Opportunities strategy, which ought to include "core race and quality standards and systems to monitor medical and nursing care audits and assess change" (p.45). The report did not mention issues of racism *per se*, nor question whether there were any anti-racist or anti-discrimination strategies in place, although these are seen increasingly as essential for establishing equity of, as well as influencing the recruitment of ethnic minority staff. Ethnic monitoring, mandatory since April 1995[1], also needs training for staff, including those in general practice, to ensure that they understand the reasons and benefits from ethnic monitoring.

As ethnic minority patients were seen to prefer Day Care, an increase in Day Care service provision was recommended. Other recommendations included a code of conduct for staff, a training programme for doctors and nurses, communication plans, Health Promotion schemes, culturally specific services which include food, and services for informal carers and support for ethnic minority voluntary community health initiatives.

Finally, Hill and Penso suggested that further research was needed to determine "whether or not the referral patterns of hospitals and GPs of black and Asian patients was reflected in their level of use of the specialist palliative care services' (p. 46). Research into different types of cancer was also needed. They recognised that community care social services provision had not been sufficiently addressed, including discharge and care in nursing and residential homes.

1 NHS Executive EL (94)77

Chapter 2

Terminology and conceptualisation

The use of expressions like 'Black and Ethnic Minority Communities', high-lights a real dilemma which is reflected in the language and terminology used in much of the medical and nursing literature in the UK (cf. fn. 1). In the United States, Canada, Australia and New Zealand the emphasis is on multiculturalism, pluralism and diversity. Referring to 'Black and Ethnic Minorities'[1] may be of value when highlighting discrimination, inequity and racism (Anionwu, personal communication), and in this sense it is a political term. Certainly, at the level of provision and policy these issues must be emphasised. But there is also a danger that as long as we refer to 'minorities' we tend to distance ourselves, and assume implicitly that both we 'British', and 'they', the Black and Ethnic Minorities, are monocultural or homogeneous (Bhopal and Donaldson 1998). This does not acknowledge the very great diversity among different ethnic minority groups, including 'white' Britons.[2] Mason distinguishes between difference and diversity, seeing difference as a problem as if "there was some primordial norm of Britishness from which newcomers, such as migrants, initially diverged, but towards which they could ultimately be expected to change" (2000:2). Terms like 'white' and 'ethnic minority' and 'immigrant' are equally "insensitive to the variety of self-conception and identity" (2000:3). This has led to social policy being determined by assimilationist assumptions, which placed the responsibility for inequality on the victims. Mason prefers to think in terms of diversity, which acknowledges the internal differentiation between categories of 'we' and 'they'.

---

1 Lalitha Webb makes a similar point, preferring 'cultural diversity' to 'ethnic minorities', which implies race, colour or religion and thus makes it difficult for those of mixed backgrounds, or those outside identified communities to find their own identities. (Symposium 2000)

2 One reader of the first draft pointed out the huge cultural gap between a working class Liverpudlean and an upper middle class public school product.

2.1. Ethnicity

The word 'ethnic' is itself fraught with difficulties (Smaje 1995, Fenton 1999, Pfeffer and Moynihan 1996). An experienced nurse told me recently, "I've never nursed any ethnics", as if she was not also 'ethnic'. Barot (1993) suggests that it is a social construction which racialises and labels the 'Other' (e.g. people who are different) as inferior, despite the meaninglessness of the term 'race' in science and sociology. Despite this, racism is real. According to Barot *et al.*:

> It is in part constituted by the persistence in political and popular conscious-
> ness, of the discredited conception of race. The sharpness and force with
> which racism persists is the principal reason why we cannot simply substitute
> for a discourse of race and racism a discourse of ethnicity. (1999:7).

The association of race with colour or appearance, and ethnicity with both, is one of the reasons for the persistence of racial thinking, and the discourses of race and anti-racism will continue to exist, at times overlapping with ethnicity. Hence, as Pfefer and Moynihan (1996) show, the inclusion of the term 'ethnicity' in data collection has incurred hostility in some ethnic minority groups. In the discourse of race the dominant group creates and imposes classi-fications on others. In the discourse of ethnicity, on the other hand, each group creates its own system of classification based on religion, culture, language, nationality and shared ancestry, but also on social relationships, shared memo-ries, and experiences, which distinguishes it from others (Fenton 1998; Barot *et al.* 1999).

2.2. The 1991 Census terminology

In addition, as Field *et al.* (1997) note, the term ' ethnicity', in Britain is attrib-uted to 'country of origin', which was used in the 1991 Census classifications. This makes less and less sense in subsequent generations, and in relation to chil-dren of mixed marriages or relationships. It also obscures the true size and composition of ethnic minority populations. The use of the words 'Black' and 'White' in the 1991 Census, creates a category based purely on visible difference, yet within this category there are people from a wide range of cultures, many with genetically and historically mixed heritage, religions and languages.[3] In apartheid South Africa and the southern United States, someone with a remote African ancestor and much greater numbers of 'white' ancestors was labelled 'black' or 'coloured' regardless of appearance. Indeed, the discourse of 'black' and 'white' populations is still in use in the US, although it is being contested in view of the growing awareness of its multicultural society (Barot *et al.* 1999). The Parekh Report (2000) refers to 'people with community backgrounds outside Britain', but this lengthy appellation will only be of value as long as people continue to identify with such backgrounds, and will not apply to those of mixed heritage who choose not to do so. According to Aspinall, "in the USA the right to self-ascription in terms of ethnic identity is considered a matter of civil rights". In Britain, however, the agencies of the state, in a number of cases,

> have insisted on identifying mixed race children as 'black' against the wishes of the parents... A few months ago the courts decided that 'Irish Travellers' are an ethnic group.
>
> The Indian subcontinent groups need to be identified by religion. It will be possible to cross-tabulate religion with ethnic group in the 20001 Census (the religion categories include Muslim, Sikh, and Hindu). The problem will be that a lot of data collections will adopt the 2001 Census *ethnic group* question (and not the *religion* question as well) for ethnic monitoring, thus losing these ethno-religious groupings (Aspinall, personal communication, my italics).

2.3. Culture

The term 'culture' is often used interchangeably with 'ethnicity'. As it does not have the same connotations of shared descent it is of less interest to epidemiologists and health analysts seeking possible genetic and biological explanations for variations in health patterns. According to Helman,

> Culture is a set of guidelines (both explicit and implicit) which individuals inherit as members of a particular society, and which tells them how to *view* the world, how to *experience* it emotionally, and how to *behave* in it in

3 There are 31 different 'white' groups identified by the local codes for the 'White' group (National code O) in the Hospital Episode Statistics for S. Thames Region (East Division) England 1995-96. NHS Executive Information Management Group, S. Thames Region (cited in Aspinall 1998).

relation to other people, to supernatural forces or gods, and to a natural environment. It also provides them with a way of transmitting these guidelines to the next generation – by the use of symbols, language, art and ritual. To some extent culture can be seen as the inherited 'lens', through which individuals perceive and understand the world that they inhabit, and learn how to live within it. Growing up within any society is a form of *enculturation*, whereby the individual slowly acquires the cultural 'lens' of that society. (1990:2-3)

Culture, from this perspective, gives the individual a sense of identity, with different 'explanatory models' (Kleinman 1986) of how the world is, of what is dangerous or safe, and what causes good or poor mental or physical health. Those who migrate to a different region may encounter a completely different worldview, which challenges not only the immigrant but can challenge the host community. This also occurs, of course, in any multicultural setting. If individuals are fortunate enough to migrate as part of a group this helps them to retain a sense of their own view of things and thus their identity. However, this also sets them apart from the majority community, causing not only misunderstandings but also prejudice and persecution. Those who have fled countries where they were persecuted may immigrate on their own, and have difficulties not only with the host community, but also with fellow nationals who may be seen as a threat, thus increasing their isolation. The prejudice which refugees and asylum seekers meet may cause them to hesitate before seeking medical help, especially if it is thought to hamper their claims for asylum and for housing and benefits. While some may be strong and healthy (and thus able to escape intolerable regimes), others have endured torture and physical, emotional and sexual abuse which they are often reluctant to admit. According to Karmi, they should not be viewed as passive and helpless but as "extraordinary people, resilient survivors who succeeded in escaping from intolerable situations" (1998:293) who are often highly educated and capable.

Cultures are dynamic and not homogeneous. For Fenton (1998) culture is one aspect of ethnicity, which he describes as a social process including language and shared ancestry. Pfeffer and Moynihan argue that 'ethnicity' will continue to be used in preference to 'culture, because the latter term "encouraged analysts to explain variations in health and disease and health service utilisation in terms of cultural pathology", which would be solved by appropriate education and cultural assimilation" (Pfeffer and Moynihan, 1996:S68; cf. Lees and Papadopoulos 2000). While the term will continue to be used, it is important to be aware of the possibility of racial connotations which can lead to stigmatising, stereotyping and a sense of cultural superiority which takes for granted Western values and attitudes to health and medicine and family as the only ones with any validity

2.4. Cultural approaches

Helman points out that "differences among the group's members may be just as marked as those between the members of different cultural groups. One should therefore differentiate between the rules of a culture which govern how one *should* think and behave, and how people actually behave in real life"(1990:4). The failure to distinguish between the *prescriptions* of a particular social group, particularly with respect to religion, and *descriptions* of real life, leads to stereo-typing. So-called 'culturalist' or multicultural approaches to healthcare (Firth 1993, Neuberger 1999a 1999b, Henley 1982, 1983a, 1983b, 1987), and in particular, 'fact-files', have come in for heavy criticism on the grounds that they reify culture and reinforce stereotyping (Gunaratnam 1997, Field and Smaje 1997, Ahmad 1999). The problem with such fact-files is that they are in demand by staff who do not know how to respond to particular ethnic minority needs, but tend to use them uncritically as a checklist. They do not, for want of space, emphasise the heterogeneous nature of ethnic minority cultures, the dynamics of change, particularly in a diaspora setting, or set them into the context of possible socio-economic disadvantage, unequal power relationships and racism. Culley believes the emphasis on culture leads to a view of black people not just as different, but as

> inferior and subordinate – as alien, deviant and pathological. 'Problems' are constructed as generated by inappropriate customs and traditions and complex social phenomena are reduced to grossly over-generalised stereotypes – the Asian girls 'caught between two cultures', the Muslim women who are 'victims of purdah'… (1996:566).

Culley does not, however, explore how to approach the woman who *is* in purdah (whether 'victim' or not) or the Asian girl who *does* feel 'caught between two cultures'. Gunaratnam (1997) argues that the simplified categories of religion and cultural practices protect the 'white' healthcarers from the challenges of death and cross-cultural interactions, but they also create anxiety about 'getting it right or wrong'. This can lead to professional de-skilling. Instead there should be a process of engaging with one another which involves risk taking and recognising the value of the client's subjective experience as an active subject. Creating an exotic 'Other' prevents the development of empathy and self examination. This process does not come easily, however, as there are anxieties about the unfamiliar and unknown, and without skilled guidance and opportunities to share the confusions, it is not surprising that health and other professionals take refuge in simplistic stereotypes, however undesirable.

2.5. Socio-economic factors

Noting the lack of clear guidance among healthcare providers on healthcare needs and service provision despite considerable research, Ahmad *et al.* (1996) suggest that it is the confusion and misinformation about 'race', ethnicity and 'culture' in epidemiological studies which is partly to blame:

> The use of these categories as independent variables underplays the significance of socio-economic conditions and health service related factors… care must be taken not to assume that differences between ethnic groups are somehow natural and inevitable and the result of cultural practices that therefore need to be changed. (1996:2; cf. 2.3. above).

Socio-economic factors such as racism and marginalisation, poverty, unemployment and poor housing, without question, have a bearing on disease, but do not explain sufficiently ethnic variations in the incidence of disease. Lees and Papadopoulos (2000), citing Marmot *et al.* (1984) show that African Caribbean men of higher social classes have a higher incidence of cancer than those of lower classes, and Balarajan (1996) found that the higher incidence of cancer among second generation Irish could not be explained by socio-economic factors. Rawaf (1996) also points out that genetic susceptibility, exposure to risk factors in variations of disease, migration and changes in environment and diet may also be factors.

2.6. Different discourses

The difficulty is that there are several discourses about race, socio-economic factors, culture and ethnicity which may all be relevant as used in different contexts. At the level of epidemiological and health studies and for service provision the factors discussed above are all relevant. But in terms of hands-on care, no amount of awareness of socio-economic factors and anti-racism or anti-discrimination training, will be enough to help nurses 'get into the shoes' of someone who *really* believes that the fate of her soul depends on a particular way of dying, or those of her son who *really* believes that he has a sacred obligation to facilitate rituals for his dying mother, and that if he does not, she will not go to heaven and will be a ghost for seven generations. What is missing in much of the culture/ethnicity discourse is an empathetic appreciation of the importance of faith to many individuals from religious communities. Even if there are cultural variations as to practice and a process of adaptation (Firth 1997), for devout Muslims, for example, there are universal prescriptions for cleanliness, prayer, diet and fasting (5.7 below). For observant Jewish patients there may be ethical issues regarding disclosure of imminent death and the withdrawal of hydration and nutrition for the terminally ill. The 'fact-files' which attempt to give guidance to the nurse caring for a dying Bangladeshi Muslim woman or Chinese Buddhist man with TB also point to the inadequacy of a training which might, at best, include a half day on a nursing or palliative care course, and allows no space to explore the rich variety of sub-cultures, religion, family-structures, social change and adaptation that are part of the ethnic minority experience. Smaje and Field comment that "much of the energy in the 'ethnic health' field over recent years has been expended in increasingly stale critiques which favour socio-economic over cultural explanations for the ethnic patterning of health." (1997:161). It should not be an either/or approach, but both/and. It is not just the patterning of health we are concerned about; it is how to give the right sort of hands-on nursing care with sensitivity and understanding of patients and their relatives who are recognised as active agents in their own lives, and it is important to distinguish between these issues. The concepts of cultural competence and cultural safety, discussed in 5.5. below, develop this further.

2.7. Classification

Much of what has been written about ethnic minority populations has been based on the 1991 Census figures, and most of the focus both in medical literature and in palliative care has been on African, African Caribbean, South Asian and Chinese – the 'visibly different' ethnic minorities, with little study of the so-called 'white' ethnic minority groups such as the Irish (Tilki 1998b), Greeks (Papadopoulos 1998), Turks, Bosnians, Kosovans and other East Europeans who may also be refugees and thus have significant psychological and social problems as well as economic and health issues to deal with (Rawaf 1996, Ahmad *et al.* 1996). There are also religious minorities such as the Jewish communities, who have had their own experience of discrimination and alienation. Papadopoulos points out that Greeks and Greek Cypriots are often excluded from discussions on health.

> The emphasis in research and in service provision has always been with 'New Commonwealth' immigrants and their families, which if strictly interpreted, of course, includes Cypriots, but which in practice has become a euphemism for the Black ethnic minorities whom British society has regarded as having the greatest difficulties in settling and living here (1998:100).

More recent migrants include refugees whose needs are not being adequately met. African refugees, for example, may meet prejudice and racism because they are black, because they are refugees, and because they have, or are suspected of having HIV/AIDS (Mugisha and Nansukusa (1998). The Somali community is also disadvantaged because of language and also meet prejudice because they are Muslim (Yee 1997).

According to the *Labour Force Survey* (1998) the ethnic minority population has expanded from 4.5 % to an approximate 10% of people who have "community backgrounds outside Britain" (The Parekh Report 2000:275); 5.75 million people have 'community backgrounds' in Africa, the Caribbean or Asia. (2000:372). In London alone, 35% have community backgrounds outside Britain, of whom 22% have African Caribbean and Asian backgrounds. If recent news reports (December 2000) are correct, the ethnic minority populations of Birmingham and Leicester will soon be more than 50%; leaving the 'white' population to become a minority. This is all the more reason for thinking in terms diversity and pluralism.

In planning for the 2001 Census there has been some debate about whether to include religion, place of birth and ethnic background. These are now being included (Aspinall 2000, Koffman and Higginson 2000). The problem with all these categorisations is that they assume the relevant groups are homogeneous. Broad categories such as 'Indian' are not helpful, since an Indian can come from any part of the subcontinent, speak a wide range of languages, and be a member of one of a number of religious faiths and castes (social strata). They are also visibly different from one another across the subcontinent. Educational levels may differ enormously (the first female Prime Ministers in history came from India and Sri Lanka – to be followed by Pakistan and Bangladesh). British South Asians also have very different migration patterns which could affect health and socio-economic status – some (e.g. Bangladeshi, Sikh and Pakistani men) arriving in a process of chain migration to work in industry, followed later by their wives, others (mainly Hindus but also Sikhs) arriving in caste and family groups from East Africa in the late 1960s (Burghart, 1987, Clarke, Peach and Vertovec 1990, Firth 1997). The latter, who were mostly middle class business people or professionals, often came in multigenerational families. These migration patterns have influenced where they settled, their economic status, the social structures of their community lives (or lack of it), the nature of the extended family and power structures within it, and their ages. Refugees, such as those from Vietnam, escaped on their own, or if they were lucky, with the nuclear family, and thus the settlement history is quite different. The effect of education, geographic and social mobility on family life and structures needs to be recognised, as the second generation may be less willing or able to undertake the tasks of caring than the older one, particularly if women are in paid employment. (Simmonds 2001)

While it has been recognised that religion should also be a factor in the census classification, used unthinkingly it can also cause confusion without the added information about self-perceived ethnicity. Modood (1992) points out the importance of religion to the self-identity of Muslims. However, if Muslims are assumed to be of South Asian origins, those from other areas, such as Central Europe and the Middle East, become invisible. He also observes that Gujarati, Pakistani and Bangladeshi Muslims are divided by language and important aspects of culture, but they share both a religious affiliation and social and economic deprivation. "By most socio-economic measures there is a major divide between Sunni Muslims on the one hand and other Asians, and... this divide is as great as between Asians and whites, or between Asians and blacks" (Modood 1992:33).

Chapter 3

Epidemiological issues

Hill and Penso suggested that ethnic minority access to palliative care services was lower than the population figures (an estimated 4% based on the 1991 Census figures) warranted. [See Table A, below.] One possible reason for this was the lower age of the ethnic minority populations, whereas cancer incidence increases with age. [See figure of 1991 statistics]. As the 1998 figures [see Table B, facing page] show, the middle aged cohort is now entering the vulnerable age for cancer incidence. The ethnic minority populations in 2001 are estimated to be around 10%, yet the figures provided by the Hospice Information Service for use of hospice and palliative care services in 1999-2000 show that 3% of

Table A.
Resident population by ethnic group, Great Britain 1991

Ethnic Group	Number (thousands)	Proportion of total population (%)
White	51,874	94.5
Black – Caribbean	500	0.9
Black – African	212	0.4
Black – other	178	0.3
Indian	840	1.5
Pakistani	477	0.9
Bangladeshi	163	0.3
Chinese	157	0.3
Other – Asian	198	0.4
Other – non Asian	290	0.5

Source: 1991 Census, Local Base Statistics, OPCS Crown Copyright

Table B. The population of Great Britain by region or country and ethnicity, 1998 estimates (thousands)

Area of residence	African	African-Caribbean	Bangla-deshi	Chinese	Indian	Irish	Pakistani	Various	White (other than Irish)
East	6	40	13	14	54	46	22	35	5,058
East Midlands	7	33	1	6	86	106	22	17	3,874
Greater London	289	455	114	58	399	641	107	336	4.583
North-East	4	3	13	5	4	41	12	8	2,492
North-West	14	38	20	21	64	245	105	27	6,322
South-East (not London)	9	46	13	18	64	391	33	69	7,143
South-West	2	13	7	3	10	118	2	19	4,648
West Midlands	9	113	31	17	196	228	125	34	4,530
Yorkshire & Humberside	7	41	14	6	53	101	112	24	4,654
Total, England	347	782	226	148	930	1,917	540	569	43,304
Scotland	4	6	1	13	12	123	24	18	4,870
Wales	3	9	5	6	3	52	3	14	2,812
Total, Great Britain	354	797	232	167	945	2,092	567	601	50,986

The figures in this table are Crown Copyright and were mostly derived from the 'Labour Force Survey' 1998 issued by the Office for National Statistics (ONS) in summer 2000, and, in the case of the Irish community, extrapolated from the 1991 Census in 'Discrimination and the Irish Community in Britain' by Mary Hickman and Bronwen Walter, 1997. Reproduced by permission of the Runnymede Trust from 'The Future of Multi-Ethnic Britain: The Parekh Report' (London: Profile Books, 2000), pp. 375-6 recorded adult patients and 18% of children are from black and ethnic minority communities (Ann Eve, personal communication). [See Table C, below] 1.16% of these describe themselves as black (African, Caribbean or other), 1.03% as Indian, Pakistani or Bangladeshi and 0.12% as Chinese. According to Tebbit, "The data available is incomplete in that only about a quarter of services provided useful information. Whether it is accurate or not is not known. Like all MDS data we take it on trust that the data collection exercise is undertaken responsibly by services." (Personal communication)

Demographically, ethnic minority populations are concentrated in urban areas, and while the figures for each hospice in relation to the local ethnic minority communities have not been published, there are indications that the utilisation rates may be even lower proportionately in areas of high concentration.

Table C.
Ethnic Grouping 1999-2000

	Adults	Children	AIDS
Services	154	6	2
Patients	48,001	212	108
		Percentages	
White	96.98	82.08	50.94
Caribbean	0.86	0.94	3.77
African	0.24	0.47	43.40
Black – other	0.06	3.30	0
Indian	0.5	2.36	0.47
Pakistani	0.38	3.3	0.94
Bangladeshi	0.15	3.30	0
Chinese	0.12	0.47	0
Other	0.7	3.77	0.47

The percentages exclude the 'not known' category.
No service recording >10% 'not known' has been included.

Reproduced with the kind permission of the Hospice Information Service at St Christopher's Hospice, London.

Furthermore, palliative care, historically, has focused on cancer, with some other diseases such as motor neurone disease, multiple sclerosis, chronic obstructive lung disease and Aids/HIV also receiving it (Smaje and Field 1997; Tebbit 2000). According to the Peter Tebbit, an average of 95 % of patients using palliative care services have cancer. However, these figures, which have changed little recently, disguise the fact that some in-patient, home care and day care services provide up to 26%, 29% and 31%, respectively, of specialist palliative care to non-cancer patients, while others provide none (Peter Tebbit, personal communication). The predominant life-threatening illnesses among black and ethnic minority peoples, on the other hand, are diabetes, hypertension, heart disease and stroke, which do not currently merit these services. There are thus several important issues relevant to the adequate provision of palliative care services. The first is the importance of obtaining accurate information on epidemiology and patient need. Secondly, there is the issue of the remit of palliative care services. Both these are discussed below. Thirdly, there is the question of access – whether those needing palliative care are receiving it. This is discussed in the following chapter.

3.1. Gathering data

In order to ensure adequate service provision for everyone, demographic and epidemiological information has to be accurate. However, information about disease patterns from death registrations has been problematic because the data have been based on country of birth and not ethnic group, which misses out on those from second and later generations (Smaje and Field 1997, Koffman and Higginson 2000, Aspinall 2000a,b). It is also not always clear whether epidemiological information is based on incidence or on mortality rates. Furthermore, many recent studies, including those discussed below, include statistics which are up to ten years old. By 2001 migrants will be a minority of ethnic minority people, and therefore statistics representing a much wider area of information about ethnic background are needed, as noted above, not least to measure changes in health due to migration. Koffman and Higginson comment:

> While the status quo persists and agencies eschew the need to collect this
> potentially valuable source of data, we are prevented from better under-
> standing disparities in health status and care provision between population

groups. *The New NHS's* commitment that access to health care is to be based on 'need and need alone' and that 'black and minority ethnic groups are not disadvantaged' therefore remains remote. (Koffman and Higginson, 2000:245)

However, establishing 'need' has to be set in the context of other factors such as demand and supply. Smaje and Field (1997) distinguish between the needs of individuals with 'chronic, incurable and terminal conditions" (p.144) and those of larger, variable, ethnic minority population groups. The need for palliative care services of ethnic minority patients suffering from terminal conditions may not be met because, as noted already, the most prevalent causes of death are cardiovascular conditions, stroke, diabetes and coronary heart disease. Secondly, even if there is an adequate supply of services, there may not be a demand for them because of lack of information about them, low referral rates from GPs and consultants, and a preference for caring for dying patients at home. A younger population may also have no need or demand for palliative care because individuals are not yet dying of terminal illnesses. A community of Egyptian immigrants in Greenwich experienced no deaths for thirteen years, and thus had never thought about issues like providing a suitable graveyard when someone died, let alone questions of palliative care, but appreciated the knowledge that the services would be available when required (Anthony Smith, personal communication). Other factors noted by Smaje and Field which might affect demand are lack of adequate dietary provision, religious requirements, and "ethnocentric attitudes to the experience of dying and individual or 'institutional' racism" (1997:159). Both the quality and quantity of service provision thus affect the levels of utilisation. Smaje and Field did not find evidence of lack of palliative care provision (supply), but made the proviso that "..there may be important considerations of catchment area and 'treatment density' which are impossible to gauge from a simple county-level listing" (1997:158).

3.1.1. Minimum Data sets

From the PC perspective, the information that is most urgently needed is ethnic monitoring of existing services, which is being done by NCHPCS and Hospice Information Service. Hill and Penso hoped that the mandatory collection of data since 1995 on the ethnic group of all inpatients for the HES[1] minimum datasets

---

1 HES: hospital episode statistics

would ensure more accurate ethnic data on epidemiology and on patient need. However, a questionnaire survey by Aspinall (2000b) has shown that that the high level of invalid ethnicity coding in the HES render the data unusable. Only one out of five trusts found the data useful, and almost nine tenths had made no use of the data, with just one stating that the service provision had been influenced by the information. The high level of incomplete recording makes it impossible to judge whether there is equitable access to hospital services. Over a third of NHS trusts felt that the categories were unsatisfactory, particularly the subdivision of the 'white' group, which should include Irish and other 'white' ethnic groups. Most trusts use the 1991 Census classification which only allows those self-identifying as Irish to tick 'white' or 'any other group', which means that the data on the Irish are inadequate (Aspinall 1999a). This raises questions about self-assigned ethnicity, and the complex reasons that determine people's choices of what to tick, especially in the absence of adequate alternatives. Local codes provided by the NHS, which do include 'Irish', are rarely used. Aspinall (2000a) also points out that between 1987-1997 only 49% of deaths occurred in hospital, so even accurate recording by hospitals would not be adequate for monitoring.[2]

3.2. Religious factors in health and illness

Religious affiliation influences health behaviours in different communities and individuals (Nazroo 1997b). In addition to the low smoking rates among Sikh men and little or no alcohol intake among Muslims (above), a strict vegetarian diet high in dairy fat for many Hindus may have a bearing on health (Nazroo 1997b). Hoare (1998) suggests the lower breast cancer rates in Asian women from the Indian subcontinent may be linked to a vegetarian diet. Balarajan (1995, citing Rudak 1994), also points to a clear link between smoking and lung

---

2 Aspinall (2000c) notes that the Acheson inquiry raised the question of limitations of death registration data for assessing health inequalities and the need to have more consistent Census, and registration data, and hopes that the *DoH's Review of National Sources of Public Health Information* "will identify the lack of recording of ethnic group for mortality statistics as an important gap in health education". D. Acheson, *Independent Inquiry into Inequalities in Health: Report.* Secretary of State for Health, *Saving Lives: Our Healthier Nation.* Cm 4386. London: the Stationery Office, 1999.

cancer in Bangladeshis, who also have the highest mortality rate in the country for laryngeal cancer and significantly higher rates for lung cancer than Indians and Pakistanis, which he also attributes to significant differences in lifestyles and socio-economic circumstances.

3.3. Cancer

Looking at cancer prevalence alone, it is possible that there has not been a great need for hospice and palliative care services for ethnic minority people hitherto, because, as noted above, they are a younger population with a lower cancer mortality rate (Smaje and Field 1997). Indeed, Nazroo (1997), writing on the health of Britain's ethnic minorities, does not even include cancer.[3] Ten years since the 1991 Census however, many of the middle-aged cohort have reached retirement. Even after taking age into consideration, the overall cancer mortality rates are lower for most ethnic minority groups except the Irish (Smaje, 1995, Rawaf and Bahl, 1998). Another problem in making estimates, as already noted, is that many of the statistics used in these studies are almost ten years old and with a growing population of older first generation migrants, the data may be changing considerably and cancer rates are likely to rise.

A study of cancer incidence among South Asians by Winter *et al* (1999) used cancer registrations and identifiable South Asian names to identify South Asian origins rather than place of birth. The study compared incidence in England among non-South Asians and the incidence in the Indian subcontinent. The results showed that South Asians had significantly lower incidence rates than non-South Asians in most males except for cancer of the hypopharynx, gall bladder and Hodgkins disease, and lower rates in females for all sites except cancer of the tongue, mouth, gall bladder, thyroid, myeloid leukaemia and cancer of the hypopharynx and oesophagus. The incidence rates were midway between those in their countries of origin and of the majority population, and were consistent with other studies on cancer mortality, which suggests the impact of migration (see below). The authors cite a mortality study (Swerdlow

---

3 Nazroo (1997) focuses on obesity, diabetes, cardiovascular and respiratory diseases, smoking, alcohol, the use of paan, accidents, psychosocial health, hypertension and CHD.

et al. 1995) showing "significantly raised south Asian rates, in both studies, for Hodgkin's disease in males, cancer of the oral cavity, oesophagus and leukaemia in females and for cancer of the pharynx, liver and gall gladder in both sexes." (p.652). They also found that young English South Asians, a substantial proportion of whom were UK born, had similar or higher rates than non-South Asians. Higher rates of liver cancer were possibly associated with higher rates of hepatitis B infection, and there were much higher rates of lymphoma among English South Asian males than non-South Asian English and Indians. Haworth *et al.* (1999) also showed there was "a statistically significant two-fold excess of mortality from cirrhosis of the liver among males migrants from East Africa, Indian and Bangladesh, Scotland and Ireland", whereas only women born in Scotland and Ireland showed significant mortality rates (p.93). Cirrhosis was higher among men born in the Caribbean, Bangladesh and the African Commonwealth except for East Africa.

A longitudinal study by Harding and Rosato (1999) among first generation Scottish, Irish, West Indian and South Asian migrants to England and Wales also showed that malignant neoplasms among West Indians and Indians from Hindu, Sikh and Muslim communities was low. Scottish females showed higher rates of lung cancer, and those from the Irish Republic, of oral cavity and pharynx, oesophagus and liver. Northern Irish females also had higher rates of lung cancer. Both West Indian and South Asian women had lower rates of breast cancer (cf. Rees 1986, Hoare, 1998). Scottish males had high rates of laryngeal cancer and males from the Irish Republic had higher rates of prostate and lung cancer. Other studies show that the incidence rates for cancer of the lip, oral cavity and pharynx, as well as liver, are higher among people born in the African Commonwealth and prostate cancer is high among Black Caribbeans (Bardsley *et al.* 1997, Wild and McKeague 1997). Lees and Papadopoulos (2000) also suggest that there is a dearth of information specifically on cancer in men from ethnic minority groups. In the United States, African American men have a higher rate of cancer than any other group, whereas in the UK the rates are assumed to be low – the 1979-83 statistics showed that 11% of Indian and African born men and 19% of foreign-born African Caribbean men died of cancer in the UK. It should be noted, however, that African American men are not migrants, whereas the UK mortality refer to first generation migrants. In the USA the survival rates of ethnic minority men are low, and in both countries the service utilisation is low.

Pfeffer and Moynihan (1996) suggest that because the cancers prevalent in the white majority group are less common in ethnic minorities, they demand less attention. Smaje and Field observe that "it should not be assumed that the patterning of cancer incidence is immutable. The fact of migration considerably complicates analysis, and it cannot be assumed that disease patterns observed among now elderly 'pioneer' migrants will be replicated in more recent generations" (1997:150). Over time, cancer rates of migrants appear to converge with those of host countries, suggesting that as the populations age and adopt a Western lifestyle and diet, there are socio-economic and environmental links to the risk of the disease (Harding and Rosato, 1999, Winter *et al.* 1999).

3.4. Coronary heart disease, cerebrovascular disease and diabetes

While there are proportionately lower rates of cancer in ethnic minority populations, the conditions that cause most concern in terms of potentially fatal illness have not, as yet, been considered for specialist palliative care services (see 4.1.below). However, they have to be considered as areas of need that might warrant palliative care should such services be made available.

According to Smaje (1995), coronary heart disease (CHD) "is the single largest cause of death for both men and women from several ethnic groups including the white population. Even among Caribbean-born women... it causes more than one in every ten deaths" (p.54). He sees the rates as set to rise. Balarajan (1995) shows that in 1988-1992 the mortality rates of CHD among individuals under 65 was 55% higher in people born in the Indian subcontinent, particularly for Bangladeshis and Pakistanis, than those born in England and Wales, but the lowest rates were among Africans and Caribbeans. (cf. Rawaf and Bahl 1997)

Kernohan (1998) found that the rate of CHD among some migrant populations increased between 1970 and 1993, and from 1991-3 it "still accounted for the largest proportion of deaths among men born in East Africa and the Indian subcontinent. The class divide again manifested itself with significantly higher mortality among manual classes, while it decreased in the majority community" (p.258). Related factors were diabetes in the Asian population and hypertension in the African-Caribbean populations. Stroke for those under 65 was highest in Bangladeshis, then Commonwealth Africans and then Caribbeans. Balarajan comments that the differentials in lifestyles and socio-economic status might be contributory factors, especially for Bangladeshis, who also show higher rates of lung cancer commensurate with smoking patterns. According to Rawaf and Bahl (1998) Caribbean born men and women are at greater risk (75% and110% respectively) from dying from stroke than British born people.

Rawaf and Bahl (1998) also show that mortality associated with diabetes is two to three times that of the general population for people born in South Asia and the Caribbean, and rates of undiagnosed diabetes are thought to be twice the rate of the general population. While there are lower rates of insulin-dependent diabetes in South Asian and African Caribbeans, non–insulin dependent diabetes is more prevalent. "Non-insulin dependent diabetes is an important cause of both morbidity and mortality in its own right. In addition it is also considered a risk factor for a variety of other diseases, such as cardiovsas-cular disease and renal failure." (1998:35, cf. Smaje 1995)

3.5. HIV/AIDS

Good data on AIDS morbidity and mortality is difficult to come by, because ethnic data are omitted from screosurveillance activities, although surveillance of AIDS cases has included ethnic status since 1989. Further, information about AIDS related diseases is made more difficult because the death certificate only records country of birth (Aspinall 2000a). Many families and GPs choose to describe the cause of death in a different way because of stigma. Some palliative care units have also chosen not to write an AIDS diagnosis on the death certificate for reasons of confidentiality, but to indicate that further information could be obtained if required. (Salt *et al.*1998)

In the UK, Black Africans are the largest ethnic group who have acquired HIV abroad with a heterosexual partner (De Cock and Low, 1997, McGarrigle and Nicoll 1998), whereas among UK born S. Asian women the incidence is rare (Ades *et al.*, 1999). In 1994-5 there were 93.2 cases per 100,000 of Black Africans with AIDS compared with 0.27 per100,000 non-Africans. According to McGarrigle and Nicoll (1998) 46% of HIV-1 infected heterosexuals are from sub-Saharan Africa but are unlikely to be clinically diagnosed and treated. For Black African adults, overall the age adjusted relative risk for AIDS 1994-5 was 20 compared with adults from the majority population, and for presumed heterosexually acquired AIDS it rose to 154 compared with non-Africans. The Terence Higgins Trust states that "In the UK, 69% of HIV transmission through heterosexual sex occurs among people who are Black, and 62% of children infected through their mother and diagnosed with AIDS are Black." (THT Website, 2001), although there is no breakdown in terms of nationality or ethnic background of these statistics. If these are current figures this suggests a rise from the 1994-5 figures. Black African children had 55 times greater incidence than in all other children combined. Because the blind testing of childbearing women is conducted without ethnic data, statistics here are not adequate, yet there is a need to prevent transmission from mother to infant.

HIV infection also plays a role in the epidemiology of tuberculosis, although cases of unrelated TB are increasing in Britain. Between 1988-1993 there was a 20% rise in TB in Pakistanis and Bangladeshis and a 124% rise in black Africans, which in 1993 was 31 times higher than in the majority population. According to De Cock and Low 27% of tuberculosis diagnosis in black Africans could be attributed to HIV infection compared to 5% in non-Africans.

Africans with HIV/AIDS present later for medical consultations than the majority white population (Erwin and Peters 1999 and Del Amo *et al.* 1996). Erwin and Peters observe:

> Issues raised included questions about if and when to start treatment, fears of side-effects both short and long term, awareness of the current uncertainties surrounding combination therapies and concerns about how to achieve compliance. The social circumstances of HIV positive black Africans living in London together with differences in cultural beliefs and experience of in the UK give rise to particular treatment concerns. These concerns include the fear of being experimented upon, lack of confidence in drugs tested only on Caucasians, distrust of the medical profession and fears of discrimination. (1999:1519)

Their study also found that refugees who did not have asylum or exceptional leave to remain had no resources for treatment, and were reluctant to start it if they were going to be sent back to their countries of origin where the drugs would not be available.

Salt *et al.* (1998) believe there is a lack of awareness for palliative care services for HIV and AIDS at both national and local levels. However, MacDonald *et al.* (1998) show a major divergence of opinion about inpatient care delivery between gay white men and black heterosexuals of African/Caribbean origins. In a hospital study, it was found that the former preferred dedicated units, where they would not feel stigmatised, and the staff in the GUM team confirmed this view. The black patients, however, preferred the general wards where their condition was not publicly acknowledged, as issues of stigma and confidentiality were paramount. Furthermore, there may have been the perception that dedicated units were where one went to die. Macdonald *et al.* were concerned that the provision of dedicated units would prevent these disadvantaged patients accessing appropriate care. The above figures and the lack of accurate date present a challenge to palliative care services, and further research is needed into appropriate provision for HIV/AIDS patients from black and ethnic minority groups throughout the country.

3.6. Irish Health

Among the 'white' minority groups, the Irish have higher prevalence of CHD and mental illness (Ahmad *et al.* 1996) and also the second highest cancer rates in England and Wales, after the Scots (Harding and Maxwell 1997). They also have twice the rate of prostate cancer. Leukaemia rates are high among second generation Irish men and women (Balarajan 1995, Harding and Balarajan 1996). Tilki (1998) describes this group as the 'invisible' minority, since the absence of a separate 'Irish' category in the 1991 Census and other surveys makes it difficult to assess their health problems and needs. The irony is that a high proportion of healthcare staff are Irish, and Tilki argues that they should be empowered to raise awareness of the "largest and oldest group" of ethnic minorities (1998;148).

Chapter 4

Access

One of the principal issues raised by Hill and Penso was the lack of access to palliative care services by members of ethnic minority communities. Barriers to access include lack of knowledge among ethnic minority communities as well as ethnic minority GPs about hospice and specialist palliative care services (Smaje and Field 1997, Patel 1999; Koffman 1997; Koffman *et al* 1999; Simmonds 2001), discrimination and ethnocentric attitudes of palliative care and health services generally (Haroon-Iqbal *et al.* 1995; Smaje and Field 1997; Koffman 1997) and religious and cultural attitudes of ethnic minority groups to services (Smaje 1995, Haroon-Iqbal *et al.* 1995, Smaje and Field 1997, Papadopoulos *et al* 1998, Gardner 1998). Tanzeem Ahmed (1998) adds negative past experiences and lack of confidence in the ability of a service to understand and meet ethnic minority needs. Several writers have raised the questions as to the suitability of in-patient (hospital or hospice) care rather than home care and day care for some ethnic minority patients (Eve *et al.* 1997; Spruyt 1999; Karim *et al.* 2000, Gocoldas 2000), which has implications for the type of service to be provided, especially if it can be shown that preference for a home death is based on religious and cultural reasons and not because the alternatives are being avoided. In areas with small numbers of ethnic minority groups assumptions are made that provision for them is not necessary (Gerrish et al. 1996, Webb and Young 2000). Other barriers include experience of racism from staff and other patients, insensitivity and lack of cultural awareness. (Pitches 2000, Smaje 1996, Smaje and Field 1997, Rawaf and Bahl, 1998)

There is evidence across the board that ethnic minorities are not aware of the services that are available (Smaje and Field 1997, Patel 1999; Koffman 1997; Koffman *et al.* 1999). Studies not specifically related to PC show similar lack of information about services and dissatisfaction with what was available. For example Lindsay *et al.*'s (1997) study on the uptake of Health and Social Services among 150 Asian Gujarati and 152 white elderly persons found a lower uptake of services by the Asians, not because of better health but because of greater family support and lack of knowledge of and dissatisfaction with what was available. The research in progress by Ahmad *et al.* (2001) should throw more light on issues of need, demand and provision in Leeds, Bradford and Leicester.

4.1. Palliative care provision

Since the predominant conditions among ethnic minority people are Diabetes, CHD, and Cardiovascular disease, the question arises as to whether the remit of specialist palliative care services should be extended to people with other terminal conditions, who are sometimes referred to as 'the disadvantaged dying' (Addington-Hall *et al.*, 1999). Field and Addington Hall (1999) show, citing a wide range of studies in Britain and the US (Addington-Hall and McCarthy 1995) that there is convincing evidence that conventional care is not meeting the needs of such patients. The case for extending HSPCS to chronic conditions other than cancer is based on need and equity. It is worth summarising this discussion at some length, even though it does not refer to ethnic minority patients, because of the implications for such communities with high disease rates other than cancer:

> If what differentiates specialist palliative care from other branches of health care is simply its emphasis on and expertise in care for those who are dying, then the question becomes whether patients dying from other chronic conditions such as chronic heart failure, rheumatoid arthritis, end-stage renal disease, have unmet needs for physical, psychosocial and spiritual care. If however, specialist palliative care has the remit of meeting the symptom control, psychological and spiritual needs of patients at *any* stage of their disease then it is less clear what might be seen as indicative of the need for specialist palliative care services. (Field and Addington Hall, 2000:38)

Field and Addington-Hall argue that professionals are already caring for many of those who are living with progressive life-threatening malignant disease in a holistic manner. Even if there are unmet needs for pain and symptom control, psychological support, family care and better communication, specialist palliative care services might not provide anything further. In addition, specialist palliative care experts may not be experienced in caring for non-cancer patients, and it would be difficult to identify candidates for such services as it is more difficult to be certain of the likely time of death for non-malignant patients. The stigma associated with cancer might form a psychological barrier to access, although it is acknowledged that some patients question why such services are not more widely available. A major handicap, however, is one of resources, since extending specialist palliative care services to circulatory and respiratory diseases would double the cost of care and result in the exclusion of some cancer patients. Such an extension would also create difficulties within the existing services and between generalist and specialist providers, exacerbating existing tensions. It would necessitate integration of mainstream health services and specialist palliative care services, which "would threaten vested interests in the present pattern of service delivery… (which) would have significant consequences for staffing levels, prestige and influence of existing services." (2000:43). Field and Addington-Hall also suggest that the continued expansion of HSPCS is a move to expand power and influence. They see the "challenge to find imaginative and innovative solutions to the undoubted problems experienced by people dying from causes other than cancer which are evidence based, collaborative with other health professionals and which genuinely put the needs of patients and families first" (2000:44). Such a perspective raises even more questions about suitable care for ethnic minority patients who do not, on the basis of existing statistics, have high rates of cancer, but who clearly do need to have an improvement of existing palliative care provision for other conditions.

However, there may be an important shift in the grounds of the above debate by the concept of 'supportive care', which is being developed by the National Institute for Clinical Excellence (NICE). This has been commissioned by the Department of Health (DoH) to produce evidence-based guidance on supportive and palliative care, and will not be available until the end of 2001. The NHS Cancer Plan, when describing the intended scope of the NICE Commission, makes it clear that the DoH use of the term supportive care includes palliative care, although a distinction between the two terms is not made (NCHS Cancer Plan 7.5). The standards set out for Patient Centred Care in the Manual of Cancer Services Standards published by the DoH in January 2001 shows that the DOH recognises that *'emphasis on survival and tumour response'* is not sufficient and it has produced a set of practical measures designed to put the focus on patient care and support alongside the processes of diagnosis and treatment. These standards are interim pending the availability of the promised NICE guidance (Tebbit, personal communication). The document states:

> There is evidence that black and ethnic minority communities and socially
> deprived groups have reduced access to palliative care services. Patients from

these groups are unlikely to take up services, which are culturally unsuitable or are delivered in an insensitive way. A total of £23.25 million has been allocated by the New Opportunities Fund for the Living with Cancer Initiative. This is exclusively aimed at providing palliative care, home care support, support for carers and information about cancer services to black and ethnic minority communities and socially deprived groups. These projects will be running by the beginning of 2001. (NHS Cancer Plan 2000:727).

The concept of supportive care, which is now under vigorous discussion, appears to embody many of the principles of culturally competent care, which would make it appropriate for ethnic minority patients suffering from diseases other than cancer, such as those with chronic neurological, heart and respiratory conditions. Ahmedzai notes that the new National Service Framework on Coronary Heart Disease has already identified palliative care and supportive care needs for people dying of heart failure by recommending that the commissioners set up working parties between cardiology and palliative care specialists (personal communication). The Sheffield Palliative Care Studies Group has begun exploring the concept of supportive care by proposing a new theoretical model which builds on and complements the model of palliative care in a programme integrating health and social care at all levels to relieve the "suffering and distress experienced by patients with chronic, life-limiting diseases and by their families and friends". An important principle of this approach is that it would provide care *throughout* the illness and not just at the end stage, helping both the patient and family with psychological care and "needs relating to information, making plans, readjustment and rehabilitation, progressive symptoms and loss of independence, and finally facing death". (Ahmedzai 2000, cf. Ahmedzai and Walsh 2000).

4.2. Communication

One of the main barriers to access is communication, with language problems being cited by both patients and providers (Gerrish *et al.* 1996; Nazroo 1997; Rawaf and Bahl 1998, Simmonds 2001). This is a problem in GP consultations and causes misunderstandings and problems for inpatient care. There is often reliance on relatives, but while this is often simpler than having to book an interpreter or arrange for a telephone interpreting system, it disadvantages both the doctor and the patient. The family interpreter may filter, abbreviate, or omit information and tell the doctor or the patient what he or she thinks the doctor and patient needs to know or what the interpreter thinks should be said. Medical terminology may not be understood properly. The use of children is totally inappropriate, and disempowers a woman who depends on them, particularly if there are inappropriate intimate details she does not want to reveal. It is also unfair on the children, who are less likely to understand adult conversations in English or even be sufficiently bi-lingual to interpret adequately or understand medical terms in either language (Bowes and Domakos 1995, Yee, 1997, Li 1998). Using friends or untrained lay interpreters from the local community is even more problematic since there can be issues of confidentiality and fear of gossip (Yee 1997, Firth 1997). Pitches (2000) observes that in Birmingham the shortage of translation facilities in the health services is compounded by patient insistence on bringing a relative with them to translate, which raises issues of patient confidentiality as well as questions of accuracy.

The issue is not just one of different languages, or interpreting and translation. Communication also involves body language, cultural rules as to what is courteous (such as not looking the professionals – especially opposite gender – in the eye) and appropriate behaviour in an unequal gender and power relationship. People who speak English with a different accent or dialect, or in Patois, can also judged to be less intelligent or fail to be understood or understand what is being said (Gerrish *et al.*, Firth 1997).

4.3. Interpreters, Bilingual Support Workers and Patient Advocates.

The question of adequate interpreting and advocacy schemes recurs again and again in the literature (Smaje 1995, Baxter *et al.* 1996, Nazroo 1997, Jones and Gill 1998, Karim *et al.* 2000). Interpreters have not just to be bilingual but bicultural (Somerville, 2001), so that they understand something about the way both the clients or patients and the medical staff think. While there have been a number of quite successful interpreting schemes, such as telephone systems (Phelan and Parkman 1995, Haworth *et al.* 1995), remote interpreting misses cues of body language and subtle nuances (Levinson and Gillam 1998). The education, culture and class of the interpreter may be as important as the language. Many interpreters are inexperienced with cancer and with giving bad news, and may not be able to explain health beliefs, medical jargon, body language, and gestures.

Somerville (2001) argues that the use of interpreters masks the need for bilingual staff and blocks the drive to recruit and train them. However, even if more ethnic minority staff are recruited into Hospice and Palliative Care, great care has to be taken to ensure they do not become interpreters at the cost of their other work. Nor should it be assumed that they can 'speak for' their culture. According to Ballard, the first generation of migrants are knowledgeable and glad to share their experience, but the later generations have "an uncomfortable awareness that their education has left them with a very limited and truncated understanding of their own traditions". (2000:8)

Properly trained patient advocates and linkworkers need to be attached to surgeries, hospices and palliative care teams. There are a number of interpreting, linkworker and advocacy schemes throughout the country, but the provision is patchy and often in isolation in local areas (Leather and Wirtz 1996, Levinson and Gillam 1998, Silvera and Kapasi 2000). There are a variety of roles, which sometimes overlap and blur into one another, such as the straight interpreter's whose job is to provide word-for-word translations; bilingual health advocates who represent the client's interests ensuring that their needs are met, and give advice on their rights (Jeyasingham 2000); linkworkers who liase between health professionals and clients; and bilingual co-workers, who work as part of a team assisting in the assessment and treatment of clients. Other roles include cultural ambassador, outreach worker, social supporter, community change agent, and health promoter, advisor or educator (Levinson and Gillam 1998). Kanchandani and Gillam (1998) also describe some linkworkers playing a quasi-nursing role in primary care, health promotion and disease management, particularly with diabetes. Despite the patchiness of provision, Silvera and Kapasi (2000) show that "Health advocacy emerges as a thriving activity" in London, with services for almost every ethnic group, in 163 separate organisations.

Overall, the schemes are largely in urban areas with large Asian minorities, and the range of different roles and titles makes it difficult to compare the schemes. The services, even when provided, may be little used. Fassil (1996) reports that in Kensington, Chelsea and Westminster, where the services are free, only 15% of GPs use them. Nazroo (1997), in a national survey, found that less than 10% of ethnic minority patients with language difficulties with their GPs had access to an interpreter. The advocacy or linkworker schemes are only useful when there is a sizeable group speaking the same language, and dangers that small groups can be overlooked (Levinson and Gillam 1998). There appears to be no study made of provision in sparsely populated areas, although Warwickshire, in their 'No Exclusion Project' (still in progress), is investigating the co-ordination of translators and interpreters (Webb and Young 2000). The Kings Fund and NHS are currently (2001) funding a London-wide health advocacy initiative. The Health Advocacy for Minority Ethnic Londoners Project[1] has conducted a mapping exercise, which found piecemeal and disconnected services. 52% of services were provided by Black and minority ethnic agencies, many of whom were generic providers. They reported difficulties in working with the statutory agencies. The priorities identified were to fund a health advocacy network, develop agreed standards for the delivery of health advocacy services, and explore ways of improving the funding base for health advocacy services (Jeyasingham 2000). A fourth priority, to provide support for the development of accredited training, is discussed below.

4.4. Recruitment and training for advocates and linkworkers

There are barriers for the recruitment, training and development of advocates, linkworkers and bilingual support workers throughout the NHS because of a lack of awareness of the need, particularly for workers in palliative care who would understand the terminology and know how to convey bad news. Low pay, low status, the lack of professional recognition or of a proper career structure are barriers (Leather and Wirtz 1996 and Levinson and Gillam 1998). There are a number of advocacy courses in Britain ranging from six months full time at St. Bart's Hospital Medical School, with GP placements and sessions on clinical care, to an 18 week (one day per week) course at the London Interpreting Project and a two year course in the Birmingham NHS Trust. A national training strategy is needed, which would provide training for bi-lingual health and support workers with professional developmental structures, while retaining flexibility for local needs (Leather and Wirtz 1996, Silvera and Kapasi 2000). According to Jeyasingam (2001), "…this needs to be done in a way that not only provides recognition of the skills that health advocates practice in their work, but

---

1 Health Advocacy for Minority Ethnic Londoners project is funded by Kings Fund and the NHS London Region. The consultants, SILKAP, carried out the mapping exercise.

also creates pathways into other related professions: health promotion work, nursing, social work, community development or medicine." A palliative care component would be a valuable addition to this.

4.5. Information provision

Lack of adequate information is seen as one of the major blocks to palliative care services for all people who need it (Pitches 2000). It is needed at three levels: information for individual patients and their families about specific conditions, for doctors about their palliative care needs and available services, and for the wider ethnic minority communities about available services. The first of these is discussed in this section and the others in Chapters 10 and 12 respectively.

Information has to be readily available in the patients' and carers' language, easily comprehensible and without jargon, but printed material is not enough because many first generation minority ethnic individuals, especially women from Sylhet and Pakistan, are not literate in their own language. Information has to be offered in accessible forms, and some community organisations[2] and primary care initiatives have introduced audio and video tapes, and used local Asian radio, community leaders and community centres to disseminate information. The increasing use of the internet needs to be investigated, to find out whether this could also be a source of information in different languages. The style in which the information is given is also important. Some of Patel's (1999) informants suggested that the 'hush hush' system of information was designed to *prevent* information so that the services would not be swamped by uptake! It also needs to be accompanied by advice on available support systems. Haroon Iqbal *et al* (1995) found that 24 out of 33 patients and carers had not received information about their illness and available services in a language that they could understand, nor had they been told about available support systems.

The Acorn Children's Hospice, Birmingham has had successful outreach in the ethnic minority communities through the provision of videos in six community languages and through visits to groups, clubs and community leaders (Notta and Warr 2000). It is "based on a multi-faceted look at provision where issues of access for all and meeting specific needs of minority ethnic groups permeate all

2 Examples can be found in the Directory of African Caribbean Initiatives and the directory Asian Initiatives produced by the DOH 1998.

aspects of the hospice service: staff, management, policy, environment, communication, community development, religion, customs and rituals and training."
(p. 148). The geographical area in which the hospice is located has a 25% South
Asian and African-Caribbean population. 30% of the total of children receiving
treatment and bereavement care are of South Asian origin, which shows the
success of the programme. Karim *et al.* (2000), and Simmonds (2001), in her
current research with south Asians in Crawley, have found that with the provision of information and visits to hospices there was much greater understanding
of the available services and willingness to use them, particularly home and
respite care. But the offer of services has to be matched with a greater level of
understanding of cultural issues around caring for relatives in the community,
family structures and attitudes to religion, if this is to be successful.

Chapter 5

Ethnic sensitivity and cultural competence

Whichever communities the patients and their families come from, they need to be seen in the context of their wider community, including their family structure and caste (where relevant). Education levels, socio-economic status, religious affiliation and faith, self identity and language all have an impact on the way people respond to illness and death. The migration history of the family is also important, as members may have experienced multiple changes, losses and trauma, particularly if they are refugees, which may add to the severity of bereavement. Social and economic mobility, as well as the availability, or lack of appropriate housing, are creating rapid changes (Firth 1997, Ahmad and Atkin, 1996, Gardner 1998, Simmonds 2001), so it is unwise to assume that ethnic minority families can or will care for their own elderly and/or dying relatives. For example, Blakemore (2000) shows that there are many African Caribbean elderly who are on their own. At the same time, many ethnic minority individuals belong to what are described as collectivist societies (Thomas 1997) in which the individual is seen in terms of a 'relational' or 'familial self' (Fielding *et al.* 1997). This will affect attitudes to care, particularly of the elderly and dying, and to decision-making, since the individual is always set into the wider context of the family.

Decision-making processes vary in different contexts, but certainly for many Muslims and other South Asians this still tends to be patriarchal and located within the whole family (Shah *et al.*, 1998, Laungani 1996). Male power roles are strongly reinforced if the women do not speak English and are dependent upon their husbands or sons to translate. However, professionals also have to take care that they do not unconsciously blame the women because they do not speak English, instead of taking the trouble to learn languages themselves, or employing adequate and appropriate interpreters and advocates (Bowes and Domakos 1995; 4.2, 4.3 above).

5.1. Health beliefs and explanatory systems

Caring adequately for patients in a multi-cultural setting demands an appreciation of explanatory systems and health beliefs, as these may influence both ethnic health patterns, behaviour and service utilisation (Pfeffer and Moynihan 1996; Greenhalgh et al 1998, Olweny 1998, King 1999, Lees and Papadopoulos 2000). Cultural and health beliefs about cancer, for example, can hinder prevention, diagnosis and appropriate treatment. Sensky (1996) observes that almost all individuals, from all cultures, have a personal theory about the causation of cancer. There are few studies of health beliefs about cancer among British ethnic minority groups (Lees and Moynihan 2000), although Thomas (1997) shows that many ethnic minority patients associate cancer with death, punishment, incurability and contagion, which affects rates of uptake for diagnosis and treatment (cf. also Dowd *et al.* 1998). For sub-Saharan Africans, illness may also be seen as due to evil forces (Olweny 1998, Lees and Papadopoulos, 2000, citing Nwoga 1994), which conflicts with the Christian teaching they may also have had, or with the Muslim insistence that it is God's will. King (1999) found that some Africans with HIV believed that HIV/AIDS was due to evil spirits or the Devil, and that prayer and fasting alone would cure them. They refused medication, with disastrous results, not least because such unfamiliar ideas led health-care workers to think of them as demented.

In order, therefore, to give holistic care to dying patients, carers need to understand the patient's and family's attitudes to health, medication, food and care, in addition to their religious and spiritual perspectives (Ch. 7). In Britain health is often seen in biomedical terms, but other cultures have different conceptions of the body which "relate to conceptions of society and the moral order" (Hopwood 1997). The humoral concepts among the Chinese, viewing health as involving continuous action, rather than a state in which illness occurs episodically, may mean medical attention is sought infrequently (Smaje and LeGrand 1997). In the Indian systems the harmony of the body is also related to the harmony of the universe. Asian dietary practices are part of a world view about health, wholeness, and the balance of elements and forces, reflected in concepts of food as hot and cold, although they are not always recognised by service providers as having a religious significance (Vydelingam 1998). Illness is related to a disturbed equilibrium and lack of inner harmony. Harmony may also be related to divine harmony and ordering. In a study of Pakistani Muslims in Oxford, Shaw (1999) shows that there may be different causes attributed to illness, ranging from the incorrect balance of the bodily elements to the evil eye (*nazar*), *jinns* and magic. However,

> Whereas the ideas and practice of Unani (and Ayurvedic)[1] medicine, homeopathy and *desi ylaj* (folk medicines) emphasise the correct balance of physical elements in the body and in the diet, religious beliefs and ritual practices emphasise the role of prayer, faith and religious ritual in the treatment and management of illness. (p. 150).

These different theories of illness causality are not incompatible, but "ultimately religious beliefs provide the 'final cause' explanation of illness'" (ibid.). A study of 128 Caucasians, South Asian and Afro-Caribbean women on the locus of control regarding illness and health found that South Asian women scored more highly both on 'chance' and external loci of control in terms of God's will, and on internality. This included fitting in with the cosmic order and God's will (Wrighton and Wardle 1997). Thus, as Greenhalgh *et al.* (1998) have also found with reference to Bangladeshis, the Islamic belief in God's will does not indicate an abdication of individual responsibility for health-seeking behaviour. Traditional, herbal and alternative medicines, which are congruent with such health beliefs, may be used; for example, South Asians may consult homeopaths, Unani or Ayurvedic practitioners, and Africans and Chinese also have their own systems of healing and medication (Thomas 1997, Huang *et al.* 1999). Anthony Smith[2], who worked with a Vietnamese community in Greenwich, noted that apart from a few cases of tuberculosis they were mostly healthy (personal communication). Because of their tradition and their language difficulties they preferred to consult Chinese Herbal Practitioners rather than their GPs. These traditional remedies may be used along with allopathic medicine, and can give cause for concern that they might not be compatible, may be toxic and lead to non-compliance if the alternative specialist advises against allopathic drugs (Shaw 1999).

---

1 Unani and Ayurvedic medicine are, respectively, Islamic systems based on the Greek humoral system, and the ancient Hindu medical system. (Shaw 1999).Unani practitioners are called '*hakims*' and Ayurvedic ones '*vaids*'.

2 Anthony Smith was Director of Studies (and Consultant in Palliative Medicine) at St Christopher's Hospice from 1989 to 1996 and held an honorary Consultant contract with the NHS as Consultant in Palliative Medicine in Greenwich.

5.2. The language of distress

The way distress is expressed varies in different cultures. Metaphors may be used to explain pain or anxiety. Idiomatic expressions and euphemisms, often linked to health beliefs, may not be familiar to the medical professionals. Krause (1989) shows that the expression in Panjabi, *Dil me girda hai'* often translated as the 'sinking heart' is used by Panjabis in Bedford to reflect a range of psychological and somatic conditions. She shows that the 'generalised hopelessness' which characterises depressive disorders in London women would not be regarded as abnormal among Hindu, Muslim and Buddhist women who would regard 'hopelessness' as an aspect of life which can only be overcome on the path to salvation. Kleinman (1986) and others (Rosenblatt 1993, Chaturvedi *et al.* 1997, Fielding *et al.* 1998, Li *et al.* 1999) have suggested that Chinese people tend to somatise distress, although the concept of somatization is contested by Waqar Ahmad (1993). Tanzeem Ahmed (1998), citing Beliappa (1991), takes the view that while South Asian patients may be well aware of their own psycho-somatic symptoms, GPs (including Asian ones) tend only to see the physical symptoms but do not recognise psychological distress.

5.3. Illness behaviour and gender

The apparent passivity of some Asian women patients, and the difficulties of communicating with them alone makes it difficult to ascertain their needs, particularly if husbands or sons insist on interpreting for them. Gardner (2001) found that this created problems for nursing staff, who felt frustrated because they wished to communicate directly with the female patients to discuss, e.g. pain relief, while the husbands expected communication to be addressed to them. There are real dilemmas here between the need to respect autonomy and informed consent for women, and respecting their situation in their particular social setting. It is important to be aware of one's own ethnocentric attitudes in approaching situations of this kind and to be ready to question assumptions that autonomy and informed consent are always appropriate. As Krause (1989), in her research into Panjabis, and Currer (1983) in a study of Pathan women in Bradford, both show, there may be different levels of expectations, both in terms of happiness and of illness behaviour, especially in public (Vydelingam 1998).

Vydelingam (1998) reports different types of illness behaviour in Asian men and women, where the men are very assertive about what they want, and the women seem more passive. But it is also important to recognise that illness in many cultures is not seen as a personal, individual issue, but is set in the context of the wider family. This can have implications for disclosure as well (Ch.8).

5.4. Racist patients and colleagues

A challenge to both nurses and doctors is dealing with the racist behaviour of white majority patients and colleagues. The issue was first raised by a GP, Selby (1999), who was in a dilemma about how to deal with a disruptive racist patient who was a member of the National Front. At the time she felt the correct response as a *doctor* was to "remain courteous and not respond or be drawn" (1998:1129), but this left her unsure of her position as a *person*. The ensuing discussion (Neuberger 1999, Easmon 1999, and Gough 1999) raised the questions of how far a doctor was entitled to state personal opinions and express values, which at least would signal to other ethnic minority staff and patients that this was not acceptable. While isolating the patient would signal that he had won, there was also a duty to other patients and staff. Gough, from the Royal College of Nursing, comments that the professional and personal cannot be separated:

> Such a position is too close to the unjustifiable notion of 'only following orders'. As health professionals our code of conduct does not allow us to condone tacitly the actions described and as members of a civilised society we cannot be co-conspirators in the systematic oppression of minority populations. To contain racism without condemnation is arguably a failure of our duty to care for all of our patients (vulnerable and captive within a ward) who are subject to the assault, as well as our duty to society as a whole. We can remain courteous, while at the same time firmly rejecting the racist's views and taking action to prevent them injuring others. Although this might infringe the individual's autonomy and right to freedom of speech and action, it affirms our duty of care to the public at large. (1999:1131)

The implications of the above discussions are explored further by Gunaratnam (2001c), who distinguishes between anti-racist and anti-discriminatory approaches. Anti-racism is concerned with discrimination and equity, whereas

> Anti-discriminatory approaches can be seen as part of a universalistic discourse in which individuals are protected from specific forms of discrimination by a system of rights and responsibilities which, at their core, stress the fundamental 'sameness' of individuals.[3]

This distinction creates tensions (or a dilemma) as staff struggle to find the balance between ensuring fair policies and trying to combat racism. A second dilemma highlighted by Gunaratnam, is associated with the emotional work involved in dealing with discrimination, and the third is "the links between 'race' and constructions of what it means to be a 'professional' in different service relations within the hospice" (2002c). Such dilemmas need to be dealt with by allowing staff to explore the dynamics of the situation and the feelings this arouses. Opportunities to examine their own attitudes and share their anxieties and feelings, as well as to address the issues at policy level, are a fundamental necessity in enabling a multi-ethnic organisation to function harmoniously.

5.5. Cultural competence and cultural safety

In nursing dying ethnic minority patients healthcare workers come closer to the heart of their own, and their patients' religious, spiritual and cultural experience than in any other situation (Ch. 7). The concepts of cultural competence (Leiniger 1998), and cultural safety (Ramsden 1990, 1993) move beyond practical skills to attitudinal change. Not only do they denote skills and knowledge which accept "the legitimate values, beliefs and behaviour patterns of people who are from another ethnic group" (Alexander 1999), which transcend language, ethnicity, culture and upbringing, but insist on empowering the ethnic minorities themselves to be involved in the development of culturally safe practice in partnership with the majority community (Coup 1996). Thus cultural safety aims to provide care which will "recognise, respect and nurture the unique cultural identity … and safely meet their needs, expectations and rights". (Polaschek 1998, cited in Oliviere, 1999)

A key to developing this is self-awareness, so that personal values are

---

3 Gunaratnam kindly allowed me to use a pre-publication draft which does not
have the page numbers of the final version. This quotation was on page 2.

examined and challenged before exploring different views (Papadopoulos *et al.* 1998). For Gunaratnam *et al.* (1998) caring for dying ethnic minority patients also involves 'emotional labour', taking informed risks and trusting to intuition. Self-monitoring, as well as welcoming feedback from colleagues, carers and patients is recommended:

> Relevant questions about the latter might be "Am I being racist?" and "Am I making inappropriate cultural assumptions about needs and experiences?" 'Referential grounding' is helpful, identifying similar instances from one's own experience and knowledge and transferring the insight back to practice. It can involve real or imaginative comparisons with similar-case white individuals or families, or to personal experience to enable empathetic understanding. This helps to identify ethnic minority people, not as others, but with common needs and experiences. (Gunaratnam *et al.* 1998:124)

'Referential grounding' is an essential basis for any inter-personal communication, because it enables one to see the other person out there as a similar human being. However, there are occasions when there is no apparent common experience. Gerrish *et al.* (1996) cite the distress and anger experienced by some midwives when they had to care for a woman who had been circumcised. This is exacerbated if the situation involves religious beliefs and behaviour with which the professional who has no religious beliefs can identify, or at the other end of the spectrum, comes from a religious tradition which dismisses all others as flawed. This is a problem many palliative care nurses also encounter when trying to provide adequate spiritual care to patients from the majority population who have a different religious or spiritual perspective (Bradshaw 1997). Thus, to interpret all uncertainty in unfamiliar situations as having a racist dimension when the barrier is one of different world views at a cultural, religious or spiritual level, could de-skill professionals and blind them to the need to examine their own world views and attitudes, or develop 'spiritual and emotional empathy'.

At the same time, as Gunaratnam *et al.* (1998) point out, it is necessary to go beyond the external differences and relate as human beings. To do this effectively means learning from *inside*, to *know* from real encounters and not just know *about*. Thus the concepts of 'referential grounding' and 'emotional work' would include struggling with, for example, the dilemma between western concepts about the rights of women (e.g. should women be circumcised at all?) and empathetic understanding of where the other person is standing – that is how her world *is*.

Chapter 6

Care

In *Opening Doors* a principal reason for low take-up of palliative care services is assumed to be that ethnic minorities 'care for their own'. There is considerable evidence that many wish to do so, but also that this is not always possible, and generalisation can result in families having inadequate support and care. Whether the care takes place in the home, at a day care centre, or in a hospice or hospital, it has to be sensitive to the needs of each particular situation, with provision for adequate interpreting or advocacy facilities and support for both patients and carers.

6.1. Care at home

For many ethnic minority families, caring for dying relatives at home when possible is a matter of honour and integrity as well as a means of ensuring the death occurs in a holy place (Gardner 1998, 2001, Somerville 2001, Spruyt 1999, Simmonds, 2001). Karim *et al.* (2000) and Simmonds, (2001) refer to the stigma and loss of face from not caring for the relatives. In the Hindu tradition, the concepts of karma and sacred duty place the family under additional stress to 'do the right thing'. (Firth 1997)

Caring for parents is also regarded as a sacred obligation for African Caribbean families (Tilki 1998). Somerville's (2001) study of Bangladeshi carers shows that all but one had some support from family and friends. Spruyt (1999) found that Bangladeshi children became actively involved in the care of the dying patient and in interactions with professionals, and had to act as interpreters. This had a negative impact on them subsequently. A number of children gave up schooling and older sons gave up work to help with care. Family members even came from overseas to help, which placed the family under great financial strain.

However, many members of ethnic minority communities are not located within an extended family. As we have seen above, social and economic mobility and changing patterns of family life may be altering the joint and extended family systems (Haroon Iqbal *et al.* 1995; Firth 1997; Simmonds 2001). When there is home care the burden often falls upon one person, but without ready access to outside support (Tilki 1998a, Spruyt 1999; Somerville 2001). Multi-generational Pakistani and Bangladeshi families who wish to provide traditional support may also be in situations with high unemployment and poverty, and large families of young children. (Blakemore 2000)

Home care is also not without problems when outside help is needed, because many ethnic minorities would regard this as a sense of failure in the eyes of the community, and it may also be regarded as an invasion of privacy. Smaje and Field (1997) and Simmonds (2001b) also point out the tensions which can arise when an elderly person needs and demands care from a female relative who may have quite different expectations, especially if the carer also has children born in Britain. In cross-cultural marriages, there may also be different expectations of care for the sick and elderly, which can cause stress and conflict.

6.2. Elders

Elderly members of ethnic minority communities are often subject to the triple jeopardy of poverty, racism and old age (Ebrahim 1996). Blakemore (2000) however, takes the view that such pessimistic perceptions of ethnic minority elders turns them into victims of racism and poverty, and fails to acknowledge that they are active agents who have frequently found ways of dealing with their own problems. While highlighting particular areas of potential disadvantage, such as the growing number of African-Caribbean elders, and older Pakistani and Bangladeshi women, he also criticises the tendency to racialize the discussion of ethnic minority needs and ignore the fact that "some minority communities are in a much better position than others to lessen the impact of 'race' discrimination, inadequate care services and social disadvantage." (2000:30).

Nevertheless, vulnerable ill elders can be overlooked, or when identified, have particular needs that remain unmet (Ritch *et al.* 1996). The high incidence of non-insulin dependent diabetes and high coronary mortality rates among South Asians leads to special healthcare needs (Rudd *et al.* 1997). In Leicester it was found that many elders had not heard about the available services "were unfamiliar with the concepts or were likely to dismiss them as being culturally inappropriate because of past experiences. Even some accepting statutory care were dissatisfied because language and dietary preferences were not being met by their current provision. Extended family support was frequently lacking" (Boneham *et al.*, 1997:179; cf. Lindsay *et al.* 1997). A small-scale informal research project (Firth 1999b) into Asian elderly revealed a considerable amount of what Daly (1998) calls 'Granny dumping', and elders with nowhere to go. However, S. Asian communities were finding it hard to acknowledge that this was happening, as it went against the tradition of family care. Lack of appropriate residential and nursing care facilities is of concern to many ethnic minorities, particularly Black Caribbean (Blakemore 2000) and Greek and Greek Cypriot communities (Papadopoulos 1998), although they might not be used by some ethnic minority individuals because of stigma (Pitches 2000). Some housing for elderly Asians is being built, but, as in Tower Hamlets, is often located a long way from where the bulk of the community lives. Patel (1999) found that in Leeds those who do the caring get virtually no support, and that in Edinburgh the service providers do not acknowledge the carers or respond to their needs. She points out that the idea of volunteering may not be part of a particular culture, and there may be no one from the community willing to help, especially if the illness is stigmatising or thought of as dangerous or infectious.

The provision of care that had the confidence of local communities could prove valuable in identifying specific needs and provide a bridge to appropriate palliative care services. One example of such care is a multidisciplinary specialist (secondary) healthcare service for ethnic minority elders in Streatham at the Whittington Centre that took time to become accepted by the local Asian community (Rudd *et al.* 1997). It gradually became established through the efforts of a specialist health visitor for the elderly. It provided a health visitor and a screening clinic with an interpreter who also accompanied patients to hospital and GP appointments. In addition there was a monthly medical clinic.

> The key elements were a health visitor with special responsibility for the elderly bringing her skills to the community, in their facilities, and respecting their traditions, along with continuity of interpreting services, a well resourced health centre and a consultant physician willing to provide the specialist medical assessments (1997:184).

While the authors do not state whether this service had links with specialist palliative care such models could provide a valuable means of identifying patients who were in need of such care, and provide the appropriate back up and support services.

During the period of researching for this review, no studies were found on residential or nursing home care for frail or dying ethnic minority individuals, although they may exist. However, the move to introduce palliative care to residential homes is an encouraging one which may meet a hitherto unfulfilled need (Baines and Hatcliffe 1998, Froggatt 2001). This is clearly an area for future research.

6.3. Day care

Apart from Gunaratnam's (2001c) study of the utilisation of a Day Care service with African, S. Asian and African Caribbean users, there appears to be little research on the experience of ethnic minority service users in Palliative Day Care schemes. Copp, *et al*, (1998), writing on day care, for example, make no reference to ethnic minority groups. According to Gunaratnam, if day care is to succeed, it has to address not ethnic identity but "individual practices and feelings about different aspects of day care services and… the broader biographical and social context in which such feelings have been generated." (Gunaratnam, 2001). She found that practical assistance such as meeting individual dietary requirements and providing transport was important, and that the Centres helped to alleviate social isolation. She suggests a "move away from categorical thinking; a critical examination of the underlying ethos and culture of Day Care provision; and an exploration of the ways in which experience of social inequalities and of exclusion may affect service relations".[1] Provision for different needs may require unequal treatment, which can raise problems of fairness for those in the majority community. Simmonds and Mount (2001) found in their on-going research into ethnic minority access to palliative care in Crawley, that issues of fairness and discrimination were of concern to the staff and patients of St. Catherine's hospice:

> Some sensitive issues also arose when interviewing patients and staff of the Hospice. For example, in Day Care very strong emotional ties had been made with other Day Care patients and a few patients didn't want this disturbed by including people that might not immediately fit in with the status quo. This presents a difficult issue of balancing the needs and wishes of present patients with a positive and fair multi-cultural approach to service provision. One

---

1 As this paper is in press, the page numbers are not available.

patient took exception to the phrase 'Fair access to palliative care for ethnic minority communities.' She felt that the word 'fair' implied a state of present unfairness which brought forth feelings of resentment towards immigrants in general and feelings that they should be grateful that they are party to our systems of social and financial support.

Some patients felt that if Asian patients have British passports they should be treated as British, and not given special preference. The fact that many of these patients had experienced deprivation themselves was seen to have contributed to this sense of injustice.

6.4. Culturally sensitive personal care

The second dimension of care is at a more personal level, and involves appreciating religious and cultural needs which enable the patient to feel respected and valued, and enable him or her to observe the necessary religious rituals which form a sense of identity. These include the need for ablutions after using the bedpan or bottle and before prayers, having facilities for prayer, being able to face towards Mecca, accepting the desire to fast as having profound religious and spiritual significance, and allowing a mattress on the floor if requested. Showers are needed, and a diet which is not just a sop to, e.g. vegetarianism, but understands something of the religious significance of the diet of specific communities (Vydelingam 1998). Space for rituals is also important – the complaint by one hospice in *Opening Doors* that there were 121 visitors has to be seen in the context of the need for the entire extended family and community to pay respects to the dying. This situation occurs in hospital settings as well (Firth 1997) and presents challenges of management both to the hospital or hospice and to the community, who should be involved jointly in discussions about the appropriate provision.

At a more personal level, carers need to understand the link between personal modesty, religious observance and purity. Observant Sikhs may wish to retain their Katchh, the underpants, at all times so that one leg is in the old pair while the new pair is put on. This symbolises chastity, readiness to act for God, and faith. Sikhs are not supposed to shave any body part, whereas Muslims may want to and this kind of information needs to be provided to carers. But most important of all is the religious passion with which modesty is observed by many ethnic minority patients. This is particularly important for Muslim women, and many Muslim men. Inappropriate hospital clothes and examination by nurses and doctors of the opposite sex may be deeply distressing (Neuberger 1999, Gerrish *et al.* 1996; cf. 10.1, 10.3 below).

6.5. Death at home

Understanding religious beliefs about death, life after death, and about how one should die, will help in decision-making about the most appropriate place for care. The important issue is for the dying person and the relatives to make informed choices and know that help will be available if it is needed, rather than to assume, as some evidence suggests (Karim *et al.* 2000) that ethnic minority patients will not want or need inpatient care because the family will take responsibility. Attitudes to disclosure will influence this decision (10.1 below), as will the availability of appropriate carers, their socio-economic situation and their own support system. As Spruyt (1999) and Somerville (2001) found in their studies of Bangladeshi carers, home care makes immense emotional and financial demands. Because of the paucity of research into the ways members of other ethnic groups approach death and their attitudes to death at home, the discussion in this section is based on available S. Asian ethnography.

For many S. Asians hospital is where you go to get better and home is where you should die and, indeed, on the subcontinent, dying patients are often returned home to die (Firth 1997, Gardner 2001). Gardner (1998, 2001), in her study of ageing and death in Bangladeshi communities in the East End, makes it clear that the home is a sacred space where one should die. Gardner's case studies reveal the importance of home deaths, which she sees as fundamentally social rather than just as individual or medical events.

> Whilst the emotional need to be close to relatives is of course central to this, there is also a vitally important spiritual dimension to such statements for, as the widows... have told us, it is at home where prayers can be said and readings from the Quran take place. In the context of death 'home' becomes a sacred domain; contrasted to this, the institutional settings of hospitals and hospices are profane, places where prayers and ritual do not normally take place. (2001:239)[2]

2 As this is a draft version currently in print, this page reference
may not be the same in the published version.

For some first-generation Hindus and Sikhs the sacred space at home is centred on the floor, to be near Mother Earth and the five elements, to allow the soul to leave freely[3] (Kalsi 1996, Firth 1997). But another reason for home deaths is that only at home is it possible to perform the correct death-bed rituals without interference from medical staff (Kalsi 1996, Firth 1997, Gardner 1998). For Hindus, to do such rituals is to fulfil the great sacred debt to one's parents (Firth 1997). An implication of this is that there needs to be an appropriate space provided *wherever* the person dies – in hospital or hospice, with facilities for other people to be present.

6.6. Community Palliative Care

Only two studies (Spruyt 1999, Koffman and Higginson 2001) focusing specifically on community-based palliative care services for ethnic minority patients were found during the research period. Spruyt (1999) focuses specifically on the Bangladeshi community in Tower Hamlets in East London. This community forms 23% of the borough's population, but between 1991-1995, 10-16% of referrals of about 450 patients per annum were referred to Community Palliative Care teams. This community is particularly noted for low socio-economic status, poverty and unemployment. The Community Palliative Care Team (CPCT) offered and provided aids such as commodes and mattresses, home help and 'night sitters' (which were rarely used), and social work assistance, although some families were unaware of the possibilities of assistance. District Nurses were actively involved in care; GPs less so, although a number of these were Bangladeshi. The referrals

> appeared to cause a disproportionate amount of team conflict and concern about the appropriate ways to respond to their needs… Communication difficulties were common, and conflicts with patients and carers frequently arose in relation to the administration of analgesia. There were difficulties assessing symptoms, explaining medications, supporting carers and addressing the many social needs which have an impact on community-based efforts of care. (Spruyt 1999:120)

---

3 Some Sikhs vigorously reject this as a Hindu custom and in contradiction to the directions of the Rehat Maryada, (a guide to the Sikh way of life. Cf. Cole and Sambhi 1978:177)

A comparative study of Black Caribbean perspectives (Koffman and Higginson 2001) on care at the end of life showed that there was not a shortage of services but fewer Black Caribbean patients than white patients received community based specialist care (26% versus 42% of white patients). While there were examples of excellent care, there were also examples of racism and insensitivity in all settings, including primary care, although there was more satisfaction with specialist palliative care nurses than with hospital nurses.

A more broadly based Leicestershire study of palliative care service provision observed that "the low level of services appears to be unrelated to the severity or nature or the disease and to reflect the inadequate provision of advice about the services available" (Haroon Iqbal *et al.* 1995). The authors concluded that in addition to better outreach and provision of information the voluntary sector could provide more social support and befriending groups, while conceding that these may not be familiar concepts to some ethnic minority groups (4.4 above).

In Derby, a survey of palliative care services overall was undertaken but did not discuss details of services offered and utilised. It was found that ethnic minority patients had lower rates of utilisation because of lower referral rates, although the younger age group and epidemiological factors may have influenced the rates, since ethnic minority patients are less likely to die from cancer than from coronary heart disease and stroke (Fountain 1999; cf. Ch. 3).

Other studies on palliative care provision do not refer specifically to ethnic minorities. For example, Doyle's discussion, *Dilemmas and Directions: the Future of Specialist Palliative Care* (1997) raises issues of care in the community and refers to neglected patients such as those with a long prognosis or in remission. He foresees changes in primary care provision and new models of specialist palliative care, but does not mention ethnic minority patients.

Issues of communication, family responsibility, financial help, housing, the relationship to the homeland, and the need for bereavement support are all highlighted in the above studies as issues for service providers, and discussed elsewhere in this document. Kai (1999) makes similar points, and shows that effective models, that can help palliative care teams collect data for effective planning, are already available (cf. Silvera and Kapasi 1998) and should be used to work effectively in a diverse society.

6.7. Hospital care

The way patients have been treated in hospital on earlier occasions may affect their choice as to where to obtain care at the end of their lives, if, indeed, they are given a choice. The experience of hospitals may be frightening and lonely for those who come from less technological societies such as parts of India and Africa, where routine nursing care and food provision are family matters. It may be doubly frightening for those who are facing death in an alien world, particularly if there are no family members who can visit and act as advocates or adequate interpreters if needed (Ebrahim 1996; Olweny 1998). Olweny (1998) suggests that for many Africans, hospitals are regarded as places where people die and should be avoided unless seriously ill. Whether one is a member of an ethnic minority or 'white' majority community, the experience is depersonalising, with new rules and lack of respect for personal cultural rules about touch, privacy and modesty (Smith 1996). Koffman and Higginson (2001) show that Black Caribbean patients spent more time in hospital in their last year of life than at home, but their study does not show the extent to which black patients preferred hospital to, e.g. hospice, although their satisfaction with hospital care was lower than the white control group. Gocoldas (2000) and Karim et al. (2000) confirm my own findings (1997) that hospital is often seen by South Asians as somewhere to get better and hospice as somewhere to die. If there is a choice it should therefore be to go to the hospital for symptom control, and to retain some level of hope.

Black Caribbeans, in Koffman's and Higginson's (2001) study felt invisible in the decision making. Haroon Iqbal *et al.* (1995) report difficulties in obtaining appropriate diets (including pork sausages offered to a Muslim patient) or having religious needs met. The levels of racism made one patient 'feel like muck'. Another study of S. Asian patients and carers in a general hospital showed that while the majority were grateful for their care, they also tried to 'fit in' with hospital culture, which they felt they were 'passing through' (Vydelingam 2000). A study of Pakistani patients found that their high expectations, in accord with Muslim values, were not congruent with their experiences of racism and intolerance (Cortis 2000). They coped with this by adjusting their expectations and developing an apathetic response, rather than risk recrimination by protesting. Vydelingam (2000) also found that the arrangements over discharge were less than satisfactory, with lack of information about prognosis and medication, and staff did not always enquire about support services, or make adequate arrangements.

6.8. Hospice

As Hill and Penso noted, there is a low uptake of hospice places, although as Karim *et al.*'s (2000) study showed, the word itself seemed to be a barrier to usage. The low rate of referrals has been seen as an assumption that ethnic minority patients would prefer to die at home, and that hospice will be seen as a place to give up hope and die. Simmonds (2001) found that Asians in Crawley were unaware that patients could have home care following brief hospice stay for symptom control. Palliative care services may be associated with a hospice as a physical place, but, as Gocoldas (2000) and Karim *et al.* (2000), note, once they have been visited attitudes changed, and once patients have been admitted to hospice care, their doubts have been allayed, and they usually request a return. Somerville (2001) also cites a respondent who had been concerned that St. Joseph's was a Christian 'hospital', but had been amazed at how nice and caring everybody was, and realised it was to do with their religion. This may be why Gardner (1998) shows that St Joseph's hospice, serving Hackney, Newham and Tower Hamlets, has an increasing number of Bengali patients. However, she also found that potential conflicts could arise regarding the appropriate treatment of the patient and subsequently, the corpse, and the behaviour of the relative around the patient or body.

6.9. The roles of social workers

Whether a person dies in an institution or at home, social workers may have an active role in the assessment and provision of care. However, apart from brief references to ethnic minority needs in a general discussion about the role of social workers in palliative care (Monroe 1998), there appear to be few studies specifically about their roles in relation to ethnic minority patients. Gunaratnam *et al.* (1998) explore with three hospice social workers issues around anti-discrimination, risk-taking and emotions in cross-cultural situations. Gunaratnam (2001a, 2001b) also explores the challenge of racism among hospital service users with hospice staff, including social workers, who are often confronted by a dilemma about their professional roles versus their personal feelings. Other ambiguities involve uncertainties which threaten to de-skill the professionals who have not done 'emotional work' to resolve the issues of their own possible racism and prejudice. "Thus, a re-thinking of inter-cultural practice, must also involve a move away from the securities of categorical thinking that have bedevilled attempts to respond to difference." (Gunaratnam 2001b)

6.10. Return to the homeland

As Rees noted in his earlier work (1986), some patients wish to return to their homeland to die, or failing that, for burial (Hill and Penso, Gardner 1998, 2001). A French study (Marin *et al.* 1996) indicated that many Africans wished to return home, but in the British literature the reference is mainly to Pakistanis and Bangladeshis (Gardner 1998, 2001). Hajji Taslim, Muslim undertakers in East London estimate that between 60 and 70% of Bengali corpses are repatriated. The Hadith says that one should be buried where one has died, so the practice of returning bodies home is un-Islamic as it requires embalming, and leaves the widows abandoned in Britain without a grave to visit (Gardner 1998, 2001). "As well as the desire for kin in the *desh* (home country) to see the corpse and visit the grave, profound issues, surrounding people's identity, their perceptions of place and the islamisation of space in northern countries are also relevant." (Gardner 1998:516). The desire to return to the homeland may be a reflection of feeling alien and unrooted in addition to a desire to return to one's roots. However, this pattern is already changing with second generation growing up in the UK and the creation of Muslim burial grounds in London and elsewhere. Research is needed into the numbers who do return to their homelands.

Chapter 7

Religious, spiritual and emotional care

Opening Doors reported that many healthcare workers commented on their lack of knowledge of the religious and spiritual needs of ethnic minority patients, and were concerned at providing the right kind of care. The following discussion shows that there is still a major gap in the literature in this area. Disclosure is included in this section because attitudes to disclosure are frequently related to religious beliefs and attitudes to death.

7.1. Religion and spirituality

While there are references to religion and religious practices, rituals and require-ments, very little literature has explored the religious and spiritual aspects of death and dying, apart from the 'fact file' type of coverage. There are a few arti-cles on Judaism (Katz 1996; Levine, 1997, Neuberger, 1998, 1999a, 1999b). Bodell and Weng (2000) explore the ethical dilemmas of disclosure and with-drawal of hydration for Jewish patients in relation to the Jewish desire to preserve life at all costs. Two Buddhist organisations have taken a proactive approach to helping the dying in Britain: The Buddhist Hospice Trust, based on Theravada principles, and Rigpa, the Tibetan Buddhist organisation promoting the teachings of Sogyal Rimpoche, author of *The Tibetan Book of Living and Dying* (1992). However, the aims of these organisations are not primarily directed towards ethnic minorities but towards assisting the majority 'white' communities understand Buddhist principles (Sibley 1997).

There are virtually no ethnographic studies of how ethnic minority commu-nities approach death and dying apart from Firth (1997) on British Hindus in Southampton, and Gardner's (1998; 2001) work on ageing and death in the Bangladeshi community in Tower Hamlets. Laungani's article on Hindu death (1996), and his chapter (1997) on death and bereavement in comparison with Western culture depend upon sweeping generalisations, but show no evidence of ethnographic research of his own or wide ethnographic reading and do not do justice to the diversity of Indian traditions. Khalsi, (1996), a sociologist, based his short study on Sikh approaches to death on ethnographic research among E. African Tarkan Sikh migrants. This does not, however, relate to palliative care. There appears to be nothing at all on the African, Chinese or Black Caribbean communities, although the diversity in these groups would make this difficult. This is a major gap in the whole area.

The lack of serious study of the religious and spiritual needs of ethnic minority communities may be partly due to an assumption that faith communities will provide their own religious and spiritual care. Anecdotal evidence from palliative care nurses suggests that it is often assumed that ethnic minority patients have no spiritual problems because "they have their own beliefs and rituals" – and once again, "they look after their own."[1] Such a view is reinforced by one (un-researched) article by a Hindu doctor (Sharma 2000) who takes the view that Hindus look after our own patients, but is unable to provide advice on how to help Hindu patients who have no support system. However, another possible reason for the lack of attention this has received could be the difficulties many writers who are non-believers have in recognising the importance of religion and spirituality for those that are.[2] It is interesting to note that Ahmedzai and Walsh (2000) do not include spiritual care in their discussion of the model of supportive care. Dein and Stygall see the lack of interest by clinicians in patients' religious concerns as due to the discomfort created by the discussion of personal matters. Secondly, they associate religion with "superstition, intolerance and persecution. Thirdly, religion may be seen as a kind of consolation, a last resort, which is offered when all else fails". (1997:292).

The attempt in nursing literature to discuss spirituality reveals the same difficulty. The current tendency to separate religion and spirituality may be of value for those who are not affiliated to a particular faith but are struggling to find meaning in suffering, illness and death. However, it does not make sense to those who are members of a faith community, and to whom 'religion' means much more than adherence to particular dogmas and the practice of rituals. If 'religion' is seen largely in terms of institutional structures and without any knowledge

---

1 Similar remarks have occurred regularly during seminars conducted by the writer for experienced nurses on post-graduate palliative care courses over the past eight years.

2 Firth 2000. This issue has come up regularly in workshops on spirituality for palliative care nurses that the writer has co-facilitated annually for the past six years. The average number of students at the workshops is 15.

and understanding of religious insights into the meaning of existence, then it will be difficult to provide genuine spiritual care to believers, as it will be regarded as someone else's responsibility. Walter (1997) points out that this makes things easier for medical staff, since the clergy can come in to do the 'religious bit' while the others "can be involved in spiritual care without probing into patients' religious beliefs and without having to reveal or even consider their own – thus the 'whole person' can be ministered to without raising the tricky subject (for Britons at least) of religion." (Walter 1997:4). Embarrassment about 'God-talk' and the failure to examine their own prejudice and anxieties about religion and spirituality can prevent healthcare workers from being alongside the patient empathetically. They may make assumptions about the patient's understanding of what is happening to them, and may not grasp their distress or their capacity to assimilate new information.

Gilliat-Ray (2000) suggests that the current meaning of spirituality in terms of 'meaning, purpose and fulfilment' may be quite inadequate for the Muslim who is less concerned about individualistic meaning than in allying him or herself with Allah, who offers peace and forgiveness in the context of the body of believers and belief. She comments that "....the idea of spirituality in the nursing literature needs to be rescued from the extremes of a) generalised assumptions about the needs of patients from other faiths, and b) generic 'secularised' definitions of spirituality as 'meaning, purpose and fulfilment'". Dom (1999), a monk in the Vaishnava tradition, who works in palliative care describes spirituality as follows:

> Spirituality is concerned with the transcendental, inspirational and existential way of being as well as fundamentally and profoundly with the person as a human being in relation to God and creation. Spirituality is normally heightened as the individual confronts spiritual pain and the ultimate death of the body (Dom 1999:87).

Such a view does not depend on any religious tradition but on the transcendent reference underlying them all.

7.2. Spiritual pain

In the diaspora setting, the established premises of meaning and explanation in any given religious tradition are bound to be shifting and changing. Religious functionaries or leaders may not be available or, because of geographic mobility, the patient may not have family or religious support. The relative certainties that would be found "at home" are no longer present and modern medicine has changed expectations of life. This creates what may be false hope, whereas in the country of origin inevitable death would have been accepted more philosophically – and much earlier (Firth 1997). Those without any faith adherence may still have existential and spiritual questions of meaning, perhaps seeking a metaphysical context for them. There are no easy answers to the anguish which dying individuals may be experiencing, and all the healthcare worker can do is to listen or remain alongside empathetically. According to Smith (1996), 'total pain' of the patient can be grasped only when good communication has been established:

> The understanding of the patient's cultural and religious heritage and the effects they exercise on the understanding of the disease process, response to pain and pain control, and their illness behaviour patterns, can then begin to be compassionately and sensitively investigated. (p.174)

Religious and spiritual people still ask questions and have doubts. Although the example, below is from a grieving Hindu woman, it illustrates the perennial question of "Why?" asked by a devout person:

> Why did God have to take him away when he was so young? Why doesn't God come and help when the person wants to live, when he is doing so many good things in his life? My husband was so religious, he prayed every day, not in temple or shrine, but a few minutes at bed time. He was a good man...
> Why doesn't God come and help when the person wants to live, when he is doing so many things for others? God helps people – why didn't he help us? Bad characters do well, why do good people die? (Firth 1997:196)

The phrase, "It is God's will" will be offered to Hindus, Sikhs and Muslims alike to explain suffering, illness and death. Ballard observes that the statement is not so much an expression of fatalism, but an exploratory one inviting discussion and dialogue.[3] The implication is that one will eventually come to see that

---

3 Roger Ballard at the Centre for of South Asian Studies,
University of Manchester. Personal communication.

it is God's will – part of a divine plan, or as Dein and Stygall suggest, "as in the story of Job, part of an educational theodicy"(1997:296). For the Muslim, peace will only be found by submitting to it gracefully, even if it is not possible immediately. For others, such a belief may take away from self-blame or, lead to blaming God (ibid).

Patients and relatives within a devout faith community might not be willing to admit these feelings to close family members or to those in the community who feel that one must always present a strong image of faith. The challenge for healthcare workers is not to provide answers or question tenets of faith (or the absence thereof), but to meet the dying person in a spirit of compassion which allows the person to feel accepted and valued, and enables verbal or non verbal dialogue to take place. (Smith 1996)

7.3. Rituals

Koffman and Higginson (2000) observe:

> For many patients and families, the crisis of advanced illness and death high-
> light traditions and rituals that offer meaning and support to them. It is now
> acknowledged that when properly assessed, heightened awareness of these
> cultural factors can influence the quality of care experienced (p.245).

Beliefs and rituals, and membership of a closely-knit faith community, do not, of themselves insulate anyone from fear of dying, anxiety about death and the afterlife, or grief at leaving the family and loss. Gunaratnam (1997) suggests that that it is sometimes assumed that rituals in established communities alleviate anxiety in a way in which they do not in Western culture, which is seen to be deficient in this respect. Rituals can also create anxiety, and it is a mistake to assume that they will necessarily be therapeutic.

There are often difficulties in supplying the needs of patients and their families. This is especially true if there are rites that have to be performed correctly. Even when they are needed, pandits, priests, granthis and imams may not be available, or appropriate for the particular sect or language group the patient represents, so that the patient may not receive the desired religious support at the end of life. This can have long lasting religious and emotional consequences. For example, a Gujarati Hindu family were prevented from giving Ganges water to a dying aunt after they had agreed that the doctors should switch of the life support system, on the grounds that it might cause her to choke and kill her. Leaving aside the issues of poor communication (although the nephew spoke perfect English), the consequences of this were that the soul of the deceased was believed to be disturbed and would have a negative influence on the entire extended family for seven generations unless there was an expensive remedial ritual. Without this she would be reborn in a less fortunate situation, and the family would suffer. The old lady's niece added, "Nurses should let the family be present when the soul leaves, because if the person dies without the family there, then that person will not be thinking of God, but of his family who were not there" (Firth 1997:123). One of Gardner's Bengali Muslim informants was devastated to be sent home and then to learn that her husband had died in the night. "Her exclusion from the scene of her husband's death by hospital workers remains a cause of great anguish. Rather than being present to pray for him, sprinkle him with holy water, and turn his face towards Mecca, she was kept separate and informed of his death by telephone" (1998:518). Similar situations occurred in two case studies in my own fieldwork, in which relatives who were not at the death bed suffered great anguish and complicated bereavements because they had not fulfilled their religious duty, as well as not being present to say goodbye and hear the last words (Firth 1997). In a personal communication, Dr. Bee Wee comments, "This can happen anyway but is inexcusable when this is due to insensitivity on the part of health professionals and bureaucracy".

Chapter 8

Disclosure

Making decisions about where to die or to allow one's relative to die depends to some extent on open awareness and disclosure. There are real dilemmas here, because the very idea of open disclosure may be Anglocentric and inappropriate for certain patients (Seale 1998, Field and Copp 1999). A number of studies suggest that in many cultures open disclosure has not been traditionally observed, and the Anglo-American practice of open disclosure is viewed as shocking (Seale 1998). There are many reasons for this: a genuine desire to protect the patient, avoidance of emotional distress and of death itself, and questions of power and control. Referral to a hospice brings the situation out into the open, and is thus seen by some ethnic minority patients and families as a death sentence, which could cause the patient to give up hope and die prematurely.

8.1. Cultural attitudes to disclosure

Karim et al (2000) note that diagnosis of a life-threatening illness is often withheld from ethnic minority patients, and staff are asked to collude with families in concealing this. In a large two-year study among patients and their advocates in Malaysian/Chinese society, Ng observed that "decision making in palliative care in this part of the world is far removed from the ideals of autonomy, informed consent and individualism described in the classical textbooks on medical ethics. Rather paternalism or power remain the prime driving forces" (Ng 2000:163). Ng reports that 84% of patients knew they had cancer and 80% wanted to be in full control of decision making. 80% of their advocates, who were mainly Chinese, also wanted to be in full control, on the grounds that their relatives were incompetent to decide but also, apparently, due to anxiety about the severe depletion of family savings! Fielding *et al.* (1998) also noted, in a Chinese context, that collectivist societies wish to preserve harmony and save face for both doctor and patient, even though the patients may wish to know (and in fact know) themselves.

In Japan there is also a cultural prescription against full disclosure, which is changing under the influence of western medical ethics (Kashawagi, 1998). Seale (1998), citing, amongst others, Ohnuki-Tierney's (1984) Japanese study, notes that "It appears that Japanese medicine and Japanese cultural expectations are characterised by the sort of 'paternalism' and 'denial' long decried in Anglo-American revivalist constructions of aware dying" (p.111). Elwin *et al.* (1998) confirm this perspective, noting that "as Japanese physicians retreat from a nearly universal approach of nondisclosure, they feel compelled to consider a wide variety of specific factors about each patient and decide whether to tell using a case by case approach" (p.1159) which include allowing for the age of patient or surrogate and the question of whether the prognosis is hopeful.

In Italy too, Gordon and Paci (1997) show that non-disclosure is not only common, but that it is embedded in a social context that believes it is important to maintain hope, security and tranquillity rather than a combative spirit in the face of terminal illness. Some physicians in their sample argue, for example, that since one does not know when one will die, to impart a prognosis is to violate "some basic order in the universe" (p. 1447). It is therefore a mistake to remove hope, which "leaves room for positive fantasy" (Gordon and Paci 1997:1449), although the authors comment that this appears to leave little room for aggressive treatment and experimental therapies. Their own research among patients (mainly with breast cancer) indicated that the latter wished to be informed of their diagnosis, but not that they were terminally ill or dying, and that they lived in fluctuating states of knowing and not knowing. Openly acknowledging the diagnosis "creates an individuation of the individual, such that separation rather than continuity and connection is lived together. It brings death into the present. Much more damaging is 'taking away hope' than giving 'false hope'" (p.1452). The aim, therefore, is to continue living as fully as possible, rather than approach death with a view to 'putting one's life in order', knowing that others will be suffering alongside. The refusal to discuss the illness has the consequence of isolating people, but it protects the "social group from the threat of separation or of openly confronting suffering" (p.1452). Autonomy is therefore not a priority: the social group is. This is similar to the dilemma in Britain with various ethnic minority groups in collectivist cultures who appear to prefer non-disclosure.

Gardner (2001) suggests that issues of control are not just ones of paternalism but, with respect to Bengalis, "... deeply held beliefs surrounding individual choice and 'rights' [which] come up against not only the practical issue of language, but also beliefs concerning the primacy of the family, gender relations, and Bengali ideas of appropriate treatment for the dying" (2001:242). Spruyt's (1999) study of bereaved Bangladeshi carers found that all 18 patients knew of the diagnosis. However, only six carers said it was right to disclose because their relative had a right to the truth and so that the patient could prepare for death. They acknowledged that the openness about diagnosis brought them closer. Eight opposed disclosure because it would be weakening, destroy hope and create anxiety and depression. Milne (2000) in a small scale study of Chinese attitudes to palliative care in Britain, found that talking about death was taboo, especially in front of the patient, and that the family would request the doctor not to tell the patient of the diagnosis.

There is also a dilemma of disclosure in the Jewish tradition. Neuberger (1999), Katz (1996, 2001), Bodell and Weng (200) show that as Jewish traditions are intensely life-affirming the question of disclosure of terminal illness presents an ethical dilemma, since Torah commands Jews to 'choose life' and the maintenance of life is a primary mandate. To disclose a life threatening illness could cause patients to lose hope and thus die sooner than they might have done. The dilemma is exacerbated when there is a question of withdrawing hydration from a dying person, as this involves disclosure, and could also hasten death. However, on the principle of balancing burdens and benefits, providing fluid might burden the patient unnecessarily, and a decision to withdraw could be made in the interests of nonmaleficence, in consultation with the family (Bodell and Weng 2000). According to Anthony Smith, while he was Consultant and Director of Studies at St. Christopher's Hospice, the then Chief Rabbi, Lord Jakobovitz, met Dame Cicely Saunders to discuss the question of whether hospice care, which implies disclosure, could be thought to destroy hope. The conclusion that was reached was that telling bad news did not necessarily destroy hope – a diplomatic and sensitive explanation was often better than not knowing (personal communication).

However, a note of caution about generalising about any tradition has to be observed. Firth (1997) found that for Hindus and Sikhs a good death is a conscious and anticipated one, and advanced knowledge is essential to enable people to prepare spiritually and practically. However, relatives resisted this knowledge and tried to control the information on the grounds that it would upset the patient. Field comments that it is difficult

> … to sensibly discuss the variety of attitudes towards disclosure among ethnic minority groups in the UK – the impression is that most do not want 'full open

disclosure' but I think that is all it is at present. The core message, surely, is that staff should not presume either that full disclosure is appropriate nor that concealment of prognosis is appropriate but – as with other patients – this must be established with the patient and their lay carers. (personal communication)

Field and Copp (1999) suggest that there is currently a progression towards a view of conditional awareness, in which disclosure occurs over a period of time, particularly as open awareness fluctuates. The danger is that this allows the healthcare professionals to retain control which then marginalises the needs of the patients. In a cross-cultural perspective it is clearly important to be aware of the cultural and social context of the patient and his or her family, to find what may be a difficult balance between respect for patient autonomy, and the need to preserve social cohesion and respect for the cultural and religious tradition of the patient and family.

It thus requires immense sensitivity in a cross-cultural setting, to distinguish between relatives acting out of a paternalistic desire to protect the patient from losing hope, their own fear of loss or the desire to maintain control, on the one hand, and the doctor's own desire to preserve the autonomy of the patient and encourage informed consent on a Western model, on the other. This will inevitably bear on the choices to be made about the about the suitability of hospice referrals if they seem to indicate there is no more hope. When bad news has to be disclosed, it is important to break it in a way that creates the minimum of distress and allows the persons concerned to comprehend what is being said. Somerville (2001) notes that interpreters, as well as healthcare professionals, need training in breaking bad news (cf. 4.3. above). McNamara *et al.* (1997) suggest that training for culturally appropriate care should include not only information about disclosure but problem based workshops on cross-cultural decision making (10.3, 11.4 below).

8.2. Pain control

Related to the question of disclosure is the issue of pain control. As Hill and Penso noted, many ethnic minority patients who are aware that death is imminent may refuse pain medication because it is important to die consciously for religious and spiritual reasons (cf. Firth 1997, Sogyal Rimpoche, 1992). Muslims may refuse pain relief in Ramadan even though exemptions may be given for the sick (Neuberger 1999). For some Muslims pain is seen as a punishment to be endured, for others a challenge to surrender to God's will. Gardner (2001) also notes that pain is sometimes under-reported by Bangladeshi Muslims because it is believed that the more they feel pain before they die, the less they will feel between death and burial.[1] According to Sibley (1997), some Buddhists may refuse pain relief in order to die with an unclouded mind. Others may view pain as due to negative karma, and believe it is preferable to 'pay now' by enduring it, than later. For many Hindus and Sikhs it is also very important to be conscious so that the mind is fixed on God at departure, and analgesia may be refused (Firth 1997)

Healthcare workers in a culturally diverse society need to be aware of different attitudes and responses to pain. All individuals, including those from dominant 'white' cultures, learn socially and culturally acceptable behaviour in order to communicate their discomfort and elicit help. Medical staff are affected by their own cultural attitudes, to, e.g. stoicism and verbalisation, and can make stereo-typical assumptions about high and low pain thresholds in ethnic minority patients (Ludwig-Beymer 1998). Bates observes that both social and cultural learning influence the physiological component of pain via the cortical centres of the brain. This suggests that coping styles can be learned (Bates 1987, cited in Horn and Munafo 1997). Several studies on pain suggest different cultures may have different ways of dealing with pain (Ludwig-Beymer 1998).[2] Smith observes that in many cultures, especially those from Asia:

> Pain is not described as site specific as in many Western cultures, but as some-thing which affects the whole person. A full description of pain may only be arrived at by delicate and polite negotiation, and so an empathetic relationship needs to be established in order to elucidate symptoms. This form of negoti-ated relationship, and the delicacy it requires, is quite alien to Western concepts where direct questioning followed by direct answering is perceived as the norm (p.176).

Pain can be measured in various ways, but verbal responses (such as the McGill Pain Questionnaire) are inadequate for assessing pain for different

1 This refers to the belief that consciousness and the capacity to feel pain continues after death, and is one of the reasons a post mortem is such anathema.

2 Earlier studies include those by Zborowski, 1952, Zola 1966, Bates, 1987, Melsack and Wall, Moore, Rodney and Dworkin, 1988.

language speakers. In a European context Ernst (2000) asks whether the 'Mediterranean syndrome' is a myth or a reality: "do immigrants feel different pain"? He notes the "profound methodological problems to assess pain perception and behaviour between people of different cultural background[s]" and on the basis of his own study, concludes that

> The Mediterranean Syndrome remains a myth. Until today it has not been defined consistently, nor proved conclusively. There is some evidence that immigrants might not feel pain in a different way, but communicate as members of lower classes [*sic*] in a different form. There is evidence that assessment of pain by medical staff is influenced by the ethnic origin of patients. (2000:125)

Research into pain control for ethnic minority patients is already underway in Birmingham University Hospital, providing "a culturally sensitive pain tool" which helps patients assess pain in different languages (Pitches 2000). This is an area that needs further research in Britain's multi-ethnic society.

Chapter 9

Bereavement

Little appears to have been written on grief from cross-cultural perspectives apart from the earlier writings by Eisenbruch (1984a, 1884b), and Rosenblatt (1993, 1997), both based on secondary sources. Eisenbruch's two papers appear to be the only study which has explored bereavement in migrant communities, albeit in the United States, and are valuable in their perspective on the changes in bereavement patterns in the diaspora. Rosenblatt's studies are based on 'small scale societies', and he suggests, that

> There are no emotions or emotional expressions that are universally present at death. Even within cultures where there is a great deal of patterning to emotional expression in bereavement, some people will not follow the pattern. What emotions are felt, how they are expressed, and how they are under-stood, are matters of culture" (1997:35).

While there is much of value in his analysis, it is often couched in vague and general terms, such as "a person from another culture" who has migrated to Western culture. It is not grounded in either anthropological or psychiatric evidence of grieving ethnic minority people in Britain or the United States. Currer (2001) wants to offer a theoretical challenge to earlier models, and cites Eisenbruch's acknowledgement that "The indiscriminate application of Western models of grief to other ethnic and cultural groups is an example of Kleinman's (1977) 'category fallacy'" (1984:324; cited in Currer on p. 52). She contributes to a vigorous debate about bereavement and the cultural bias or culture-blindness that has been displayed in many earlier studies. Field, Hockey and Small (1997) view critically the psychoanalytic or psychodynamic approach, which

> … assumes that individual behaviour is based upon the early shaping of biological needs and drives which remain basically unaltered throughout a person's life… Explanations of their reactions to illness, dying and the death of another are to be sought within the experiencing individual rather than in the social contexts and social relationships within which these experiences occur. (p.24)

They describe this as influential model ethnocentric, determinist, individualist and masculinist in its approach, although they do not take the analysis further in relation to a multicultural perspective on bereavement. A more inter-actionist approach allows for the influence of social contexts, placing "particular emphasis on communication and meaning and how these affect the experiences of (dying) patients, their relatives and others close to them, and those caring for them" (p.23). However, these have been limited in their application, and "rarely address the effect of broader social constraints, such as political and economic structures." (ibid).

A recognition of cultural differences is shown by Stroebe and Schut (1998), who criticise "Western concepts of 'normal reactions' or 'healthy' ways of coping... as ethnocentric constructions" (cited in Currer 2001:53). They acknowledge, as Rosenblatt and Eisenbruch did before them, that cultural vari-ations are influenced by the prescriptions of a particular society. They propose a 'dual process' model of grieving, in which at times there is an orientation towards loss, to 'letting go of the past', and at other times an orientation towards restora-tion, to remaining with or keeping hold of the deceased. This model allows for cultural variations, such as the reconstruction of the deceased as an ancestor (below), as well as other factors that influence grief.

Another critic of contemporary approaches is Walter. His arguments are particularly useful for throwing light on cross-cultural perspectives on bereave-ment and will be drawn on for the discussion, below. In what he describes as "an over-neat formulation", he distinguishes between bereavement as "the objective state of having lost someone or something, grief [as] the emotions that accom-pany bereavement" and "Mourning [as] the behaviour that social groups expect following bereavement" (1999:xv). Grief, he argues, is as subject to cultural influences as bereavement and mourning, and that includes variations in the 'majority' American and British culture's approaches to bereavement. Of partic-ular importance in Walter's 'New Model of Grief' (1996) is its location in the social sphere, recognising the need to talk through the narrative of the death with others who shared knowledge of the deceased person:

> Bereavement... is the state of being caught between the present, a past and a lost future. Rewriting the past to make sense of the new present is crucial if sense is to be made of change and the future faced.... Telling the story of the lost one and how they were lost, going over it with others as well as in one's own head, is a typical experience of bereavement, especially if the death was unexpected. Only then can survivors begin to get a handle on their new situa-tion. (1999:70)

In the Jewish *shiva* the seven days of sitting provide opportunities to go over and over the event, and in the S. Asian communities, friends, relatives and neighbours come and sit daily for ten or more days, again providing opportunities to talk about the deceased and what happened when the death occurred. Shared narratives about the person and about the death help to recreate the person in people's minds, while the shared stories about other people's bereavements place the death in a context of universal experience.

Walter recognises the importance of religious belief and practice in coping with bereavement, commenting that "The role of prayer in bereavement is distinctly under-researched" (p.59). He cites examples of people who talked to God, or "created for themselves spiritual imagery". He makes an important distinction between the roles of therapy and religion, illustrated by the example of a woman who sought help from spiritualists for assurances that her dead mother was at peace (the role of religion), rather than help for herself (the role of therapy). Currer also sees a link between religious beliefs and the response to illness and death, which recognises that grieving is in part about the meanings which people attribute to life and death. "It is perhaps only surprising that some theoreticians insist upon the universality of the emotional processes of grief, in the face of apparently contradictory beliefs about the implications of dying (total extinction or the gateway to something better, for example)". (2001:55).

For South Asians the mourning period provides a context for placing death and suffering within a shared framework of religious meaning, with readings from the texts, hymn singing and little homilies by senior members of the community. This involves making sense of the death by trying to find ways to explain it in terms of God's will, heaven, and for Hindus and Sikhs, rebirth. Attempts are made to view the death as a 'good death', even in the face of evidence to the contrary, which provides some consolation. For example, when a 72 year-old Hindu man had a heart attack in his doctor's surgery, the suddenness of the death and possible pain indicated that he had had a bad death. However, the fact that the Hindu doctor cradled the dying man in is arms and told him to repeat the name of God was cited as evidence that it was a good death (Firth 1997). Subsequently his wife struggled to find meaning in his death and found it in the shared stories about other people's bereavements, which placed her own experience within a universal context, and in the teaching of the *Bhagavad Gita:*

> Sometimes when I am alone I think, "Oh, that is a life now, the children were here, now I am alone, what about me?" Then I think, the *atma* (soul) is

eternal, he has gone and my turn is coming. I pray to God, my body is yours, my husband's body was yours, my children's bodies. Who is dead? Nobody is dead if you believe the atma is eternal. Everyone's turn will come, and when my turn comes my children will miss me, as we miss our parents, but in *samsar* (the cycle of birth and death) it is like this, and then you have peace. When you read (*The Bhagavad Gita*) this reminds you that we change our bodies, like clothes, and we have a new birth. People come and go, come and go, and you think, my parents have died, others have died… then (the people who come to visit) say, "my son has died, my daughter has died", and share with you. In every house death has come. Then you have peace (Firth 1997, adapted).

Following Klass (1997), Walter (1999) also recognises the importance of making or creating a place for the dead. Although for Walter this is done in part by talking about the deceased, thus locating them in a societal context, he also recognises the importance of religious beliefs, recognising the validity of people's experiences of the presence of the dead and the importance of objects such as the grave, photographs and mementoes. In many earlier studies (Rees 1971, Parkes 1972), visions or awareness of the deceased have been given a reductionist explanation in terms of 'hallucinations'. Western Protestant culture has tried to 'get rid of the dead', so that the funeral is the end of the matter – there is no on-going relationship with them. Walter recognises the importance of 'bringing them back' into the family, in one form or another, so that they "exist not only internally within the head of a bereaved individual but are also (as any member of an ancestor venerating tribe could tell us) communally constructed within groups" (1999: 191). The creation of the deceased as an ancestor, who will then remain in a symbiotic relationship with the living, is common in many ethnic minority cultures in Britain, including Hindu, Chinese and African societies. For Hindus, during the mourning period, the body of the deceased is ritually recreated, and in a powerful ceremony on the twelfth day, is 'sent off' as an ancestor (Firth 1997). No literature was found during the research period on British Chinese rituals, but a British Chinese anthropologist, Thornhill-Lee, describes the prayers and rituals for a Singapore Chinese funeral which "transform the deceased from a dangerous and polluting spirit to a settled and benevolent ancestor" (2000). For both Hindus and Chinese, the belief that the spirit is dangerous and polluting until the appropriate rituals have been completed has important implications for bereavement support, since it is important for those who provide the support to recognise in a non-judgemental way the anxiety associated with such beliefs. Once the rituals have been completed, the ancestors remain in a symbiotic relationship with the family, providing progeny, health and wealth in exchange for gifts and honour.

Social position is also relevant to grief and mourning. Currer suggests that those who are powerless, such as the Pathan women she studied (1986) are more vulnerable if they have no sense of control over events and grief. There is often a dramatic change of social and socio-economic status and stigma for Hindu and Sikh widows. They are particularly vulnerable, if they have no sons, and support for them cannot be taken for granted. Older Hindu widows may also face social exclusion in more traditional caste groups, which is often accompanied by a loss of a sense of self-worth and meaning. This is because the failure to die before one's husband implies either that one has bad karma from a previous life, or has failed to keep him alive by the appropriate rituals (Firth 1999a). A traditional Hindu widow would be expected to continue mourning her husband for the rest of her life and to withdraw from normal social intercourse because she is unlucky and impure. One Hindu widow in Britain, in her 50s internalised traditional attitudes to widows to such an extent that she did not go out of her house for ten years (Firth 1997). British Bengali Muslim widows are more likely than most to experience poverty and isolation if they do not have a support system, especially if they do not speak English. To visit the grave of the deceased is particularly important in Islam. However, if the body is returned to Bangladesh for burial and she cannot go because of the cost, she may feel she has failed in her obligation to her husband (Gardner 1998). The creation of Muslim cemeteries in London and elsewhere is likely to change this, particularly if there are adult children who wish to have the burial in this country so that they can visit the grave.

9.1. Grief Behaviour

Hill and Penso mention the difficulties for staff of many relatives weeping around a deathbed, and one of Gardner's nurse informants refers to "30 or more people 'screaming' around the bed" (1998:515). Quite apart from the disruption this causes, the comments reveal considerable discomfort for people from a traditionally British 'stiff upper lip' society in dealing with a more extroverted and noisy expression of grief. Dr. Bee Wee comments that the professsionals' own discomfort can be hidden behind the claim that "We have to consider other patients" (personal communication).

Walter (1999) distinguishes between expressive and non-expressive cultures. Among the former he includes Italy, Ireland, Greece and Orthodox Judaism. These 'ritualize emotion in a way that would embarrass most English' (p.139). By contrast Scotland, England, Germany, Switzerland, Finland Australia, the Netherlands and parts of the USA discourage public expressions of emotion. However, Walter points to the range of patterns of grief within 'English' society as well as expressive British ethnic minority groups such as Irish (Catholic, working class) Caribbean, Muslim (female), Hindu, and Orthodox Jewish. He hastens to add that this does not mean stereotyping, but a pointer to variations of grief behaviour within as well as between cultural groups. In a hospice or hospital context some understanding of these variations as completely normal within a particular group's expectations might help in dealing with the real dilemmas presented by expressive grief on a ward, by, for example, providing appropriate space for the relatives and other mourners. Bahl (1996), commenting on the need to express grief in culturally appropriate ways, observes:

> Many black and minority ethnic people may also wish to rely on the thera-
> peutic value of the expression of strong emotions and the supportive grieving
> of others concerned to help them come to terms with loss. If these issues are
> not appreciated by service providers, however, then being denied the very
> coping mechanisms traditionally adopted by these communities could result in
> added distress for those dying, or bereaved... Many minority ethnic people
> who are bereaved may not feel able to openly express their anxieties and
> emotions for fear of not being understood by health workers who may appear
> to hold a different set of beliefs and values. (p.57)

9.2. Bereavement support

Hill and Penso and Spruyt (1999) refer to the need for bereavement support for ethnic minority relatives. It cannot be assumed that even in closely-knit communities there will be adequate support after the death, particularly if the patient has died of a stigmatising disease. A young Hindu widow, for example, may be blamed by her husband's family for his premature death, and if she has no kin of her own in Britain she can be very isolated (Firth 1999a). Blakemore (2000) refers to the social isolation of many elderly African Caribbeans, and the spouse of an elderly person in any community may have no support at all. The way in which the family member died, the circumstances of the death, experiences of misunderstanding and racism can all complicate bereavement. Koffman and Higginson (2001), referring to African-Caribbean carers, noted that "not experiencing bereavement-related psychological problems is associated with high satisfaction of services by caregivers" – in other words, those that were not satisfied with the services were more likely to suffer bereavement-related problems. In particular, those ethnic minority bereaved who have failed to meet religious requirements, or fulfill what they consider to be their duty, will not only suffer greater problems after the death, but need support which accepts and understands their anxieties. Further, those Hindus whose relatives have had a 'bad death' (Firth 1997) may be intensely anxious about the ghost of the deceased, and anyone offering support has to accept this world view without judgement so that the feelings can be shared.

Careful thought has to be given as to the nature of bereavement support. Field (personal communication) notes that there is a debate about the efficacy of counselling among care providers, some of whom question its use for bereavement support. The role of the bereavement counsellor, according to Walter, is "to provide a safe place where feelings can be expressed and accepted, and to assure the client that these feelings are normal and that he or she is not going mad" (1999:197). He distinguishes between those therapies emphasising resolution, such as psychodynamic, which imply there is a time at which the client has resolved his or her grief and 'let go'; and those which see grief as a process in which the counsellor helps to bereaved to edit or clarify their chaotic feelings. "The product is an account, existing outside of themselves, which the bereaved person then submits to further processes of interpretation" (Hockey 1986:334, cited in Walter 1999:198). There are thus various approaches which range from the prescriptive, which provide a map of grief, such as the stages theory (Kübler-Ross 1970, 1975) or Worden's (1991) tasks of grief, those that move towards integration, or those that help provide a setting in which the dead continues to exist, such as the Compassionate Friends.

However, bereavement support, while it requires training in some counselling and listening skills, is not intended to be therapy or counselling. If it is to be offered to ethnic minority families and individuals, there must be adequate and appropriate training which enables the supporter to grasp the complexities of the cultural context in which the bereaved individual finds him or herself. Training for bereavement support, as with culturally competent nursing training, has to enable the supporter to lay aside his or her own cultural expectations and be willing to enter that of the client. If individuals from the majority community provide bereavement support, it is particularly important to accept different gender roles, and not allow Western expectations of autonomy and independence to affect judgement of women clients. It is important also to recognise cultural issues and conflicts, which may emerge as the client confronts the life changes ahead. Walter (1999) notes such conflicts in bereavement are not uncommon. Citing Shapiro (1994, 1996), who from "an American context strongly influenced by immigration and inter-ethnic marriage" he suggests that the way in which a person wishes to grieve may not meet the "cultural expectations and required rituals of their family and community". The therapist or supporter's role is "to help the client explore the goodness of fit between personal style and group experience". Those who have settled in a new country may find issues from the country of origin resurfacing at such times, especially if they have married someone from another community. "This is particularly likely if the deceased had a symbolic significance in the drama of immigration" (p.152). People living in the diaspora may have fragile identities when uprooted from their home and culture, and the loss of a loved person, especially a husband or parent, threatens the sense of who one is. In addition, many first generation migrants have experienced multiple losses, of home, country and even, for those who are twice or thrice migrants, more than one country. The second generation have to make sense of this, especially if they have married 'out' of their ethnic group.

Ideally members of the respective communities will undergo training for bereavement support. A Muslim Bereavement Service[1] is being established by the City and East London Bereavement Counselling service, which aims to train Muslims to be bereavement visitors. However, the visitors will have a wider role giving advice when required, making appropriate referrals and acting as advocates. This has been set up in partnership with the local Bangledshi community, members of which are serving on the steering committee (Jan Fish, personal communication).

1 The Muslim Bereavement Service is funded by the National Lottery and Kings Fund

Chapter 10

The medical profession

General practitioners, as has been noted above, and hospital consultants play a crucial role in ensuring ethnic minorities obtain adequate health care, and as Hill and Penso suggest, act as gatekeepers to palliative care services. If sick patients are not being referred it is important to ascertain the reasons. There are two possible problems here – lack of awareness of hospice and specialist palliative care services, and lack of knowledge of the local minority ethnic populations. An assumption that patients 'care for their own' (6.1 above) is not borne out by the evidence, although equally, it is clear that many families wish to do so. However, if the doctors serving the local community are unaware of local circumstances and know nothing about the local communities in all their rich variety, they will not be able to make appropriate referrals or arrange for the most suitable care.

10.1 GP services

Hill and Penso, and Karim *et al.* (2000) raise questions as to whether ethnic minority patients are being offered an adequate range of choices with regard to palliative care services, or understand what they are when they are made available (Haroon Iqbal *et al.* 1995). Patients and their doctors may have major communication problems, so that the doctor is unable to ascertain the needs and wishes of the sick person and their relatives. A GP without an understanding of different cultural traditions may have difficulties over issues of disclosure (above) if the patient's family wish to conceal the diagnosis and/or prognosis, which makes referrals more difficult. Koffman and Higginson's (2001) study of Black Caribbeans in the last year of life showed that there was lower satisfaction with primary care than with acute care, possibly because of the difficulty of providing adequate services in deprived inner-city areas. As they also found, many ethnic minority patients feel they are not given enough time, taken seriously enough or examined properly (cf. Fassil 1996, Yee 1997). Nazroo (1997) suggests that less than 10% of GPs have professional interpreters or advocates during consultations. In a study of four groups of service users (Black Caribbean, Asian, Chinese and Somali) by the RCGP (Yee 1997), racism was shown to be a major factor in the way the Black Caribbean group and Somalis were treated. Yee's study found that because of a reluctance to use GPs there is greater use of A&E for what may be considered to be trivial complaints (Yee 1997). Although there is some indication that Asian patients show higher GP consultation rates than the majority population (McCormick, Fleming and Charlton, 1995, Chaturvedi *et al* 1997), Kai (1999) comments that more consultations do not mean better care, or effective or appropriate care, and the low rates of referrals may reflect this (Chaturvedi *et al* 1997).

Dissatisfaction with GPs, or anxiety about consultations, could also have a bearing on late presentation for cancers and HIV/AIDS, in addition to stigma. A reluctance to be examined by male doctors for religious and cultural reasons may also be a reason for late presentation of gynaecological conditions or breast cancer by some ethnic minority women (Ahmad *et al* 1989, Bowes and Domokos 1995, Bhakta *et al*. 1995,Bahl 1996). Smaje (1995) suggests that the research evidence that South Asian women would prefer to consult a female doctor is inconclusive, as some women appear to prefer an Asian GP who speaks the same language (Pilgrim *et al.*, 1993, Raschid and Jagger 1992). However, even if an ethnic minority woman was willing to *consult* a male doctor from the same culture, she may be hesitant to be *examined* by him (Nazroo 1997). Papadopoulos (1998) makes the same point about Greek women – they would refuse a smear test, for example, unless a woman did it. Bahl (1996) found that the uptake for both breast and cervical screening was lower for South Asian women, and Papadopoulos indicates that there are similar issues for other ethnic minority women.

10.2. Referrals

Are doctors encouraging or preventing access? Low referral rates continue to be seen as a problem (Koffman 1998, Gerrish 1999). Rees found in his 1986 study of St. Mary's Hospice that while the referral rates for palliative care were lower (3.6% average), the uptake of referrals was higher than with white patients. In a study of the referrals of 12 GPs and 15 hospital consultants to the same hospice in Birmingham, Karim *et al.* (2000) found an increase in the ethnic minority referral rate in 1996-1997 to 8.5%, and also showed there was a high uptake, but that this was still not commensurate with the size of the local population. One reason for not making referrals was that the doctors believed ethnic minority families preferred to provide palliative care themselves, although they admitted this was based on impressions with no empirical basis. Unfortunately Karim *et al.* do not give details about how many of these were themselves from ethnic minority communities, or indicate which doctors made particular observations. If it could be shown, as some evidence suggests, that Asian or other ethnic minority doctors were referring fewer ethnic minority patients to palliative care, it is most important that the reasons be ascertained, especially if this is because they are unaware of PC services.

If, as Alexander shows, 20% of Indian, 50% of Pakistani and 59% of Bangladeshis communicate with their GPs in an Asian language, the referral rates of Asian GPs need further investigating. Ethnic minority doctors are no more homogeneous as a group than the communities they serve, and they may be making unjustifiable assumptions about patients from different or lower caste backgrounds based on an ideal model of the community, or based on western medical models. Chaturvedi *et al.* (1997) also point out that many ethnic minority doctors are trained according to the 'Western cultural paradigm' and may not be familiar with traditional or alternative systems, or indeed with different ethnic minority communities. Somerville (2001) reports that Bangladeshi patients in her study received minimal contact with their GPs during their final illness, although they received nursing support.

For those patients needing in-patient hospice care at the end stage of their disease, Ahmedzai (personal communication) suggests that there may already be an element of selection taking place. For example, Addington Hall et al. (1998) found patients with cancer who were admitted to hospices were younger than those with cancer who were not admitted. Younger women with, e.g. breast cancer, may be more likely to be referred for care than older men with prostate cancer who may not demand such care. If hospices do not take all patients in strict proportion to their diagnosis then there is already an in-built bias where referrals are concerned, and as the discussion (4.1) above, indicates, there are arguments for extending palliative care to ethnic minority patients suffering from diseases other than cancer.

According to Gerrish (1999), a serious issue for equitable palliative care services is the inequitable allocation of district nursing resources to GPs. She found that single-handed inner-city doctors with big ethnic minority populations received much smaller allocations of staff than single group practices with smaller white populations. However, she also found that those who were referred for nursing care received it.

10.3. The experience of caring for ethnic minority patients

In *Opening Doors* it is evident that nurses were anxious about nursing ethnic minority patients, and felt unsure about communication, gender issues, disclosure policies, and their own lack of understanding about cultural practices. These are also issues for medical practitioners. Conscious and unwitting racism, exemplified by stereoptying and generalising, ignorance about different cultures and religions, and ethnocentric attitudes to different behaviours have all been reported by patients and clients. Yet patients from any community should be able to receive holistic palliative care at the end of life. Appropriate training in cultural competence is needed, at both undergraduate and post-graduate or in-service levels which aims not just at an increase in information and knowledge but attitudinal changes leading to greater understanding and empathy. This will improve care to all patients, regardless of ethnicity, religion or cultural background.

Murphy and McLeod Clark (1993) looked at nurses' perceptions of caring for ethnic minority patients in hospital. They found that "In some cases communication was so poor it was impossible to identify individual client problems at all" (p.449). Such difficulties created negative feelings, causing nurses to distance themselves from the patients. Many found the situation stressful, and tended to focus on tasks and routines, which contradicted the palliative care goal of holistic care. Many of the nurses had "ethnocentric beliefs about the superiority of Western health standards [and] little apparent understanding by respondents of illness behaviour" (ibid.). Gunaratnam (2001c) also found anxiety, uncertainty and ambivalence in her research in a hospice, which she suggests were exacerbated by the palliative care environment. Nurses were particularly afraid to take risks in case they 'got it wrong': "others deliberated about the validity of their perceptions of cultural phenomena, while others talked about the difficulties of managing inter-cultural differences between service users". One nurse refers to her difficulty of communicating with an African patient:

> I found it extremely hard to get alongside her, I would say because of the
> cultural differences… there was a lot to her case in particular, but I found it
> with Ugandan women in particular… to I suppose read them… I suppose I go

a lot on peoples' non-verbals as well as what they say, and when the language is different you go a lot on peoples' non-verbals... I suppose I view that as a failure of care in a way... but then, can we ever, as somebody from a different culture... could I ever have done that given more time?" [1]

Some of Gunaratnam's informants felt that "Formal commitments to multi-culturalism and equal opportunities can sometimes actually make it more diffi-cult for staff to explore and to ask for help around areas of ambiguity in practice because 'it would be a bit like identifying yourself as having racist tendencies.'"

Gunaratnam sees "attention to difference... as an integral part of holistic care." However, despite a commitment to holistic care and to addressing multi-cultural issues, she found in her research that "there was often an inadequate understanding amongst staff about the ways in which ethnicity, and social inequalities in particular, could affect palliative care needs." Individuals' experi-ences of racism and discrimination were often "neglected by the inability or unwillingness of practitioners to provide specific recognition and support for the ways in which social inequalities, such as racism, can effect disease, physical, emotional and spiritual pain and caring relationships." She gives the example of a Jamaican woman who had experienced both domestic and racist abuse, who was thought by nurses to be 'anxious' and 'paranoid', yet described being washed by nurses as being frightening. She felt "objectified 'like a piece of meat'". The desire to 'go home' to die or for burial was assumed by some healthcare workers to be a 'cultural' issue, whereas Gunaratnam found that "these representations were also often powerful emotional and social commentaries that not only entailed negotiating dimensions of cultural identity, but also involved more generalised feelings of belonging, loss and separation". Labelling issues as 'cultural' served the purpose of distancing or 'Othering', but also marked out 'no-go areas' for care.

10.4. Education of medical professionals

The evidence of low referral rates and dissatisfaction with GPs and hospital doctors suggests that for effective palliative care services the medical profes-sionals need more interdisciplinary education about ethnic minority communi-ties during medical training, as well as during postgraduate training for general

---

1 As these quotations are taken from a prepublication draft, page numbers are unavailable.

practice and palliative medicine. However, no literature was found which examined the attitudes of doctors in either general practice or palliative medicine, to ethnic minority patients needing palliative care, apart from Karim *et al.*'s (2000) limited study on referrals. This, as has been noted, suggests both a stereotypical view of ethnic minority requirements and lack of awareness of palliative care services. Broadening the understanding of doctors especially in primary care and in palliative medicine, about ethnic minorities and introducing the principles of cultural competence would make doctors more sensitive and benefit all patients.

Of relevance to caring for ethnic minority patients is a new resource commissioned by the RCGP that aims to introduce valuing ethnic diversity into health education with a training pack and video. This offers practical suggestions on culture, working with trained interpreters or advocates, and placing the needs of ethnic minorities in context (Yee 1997, Kai 1999). Other issues raised include encouraging research and teaching about appropriate touch, listening skills and non-verbal communication. Training on racism awareness should include understanding the status of refugees and ways to treat black patients in a culturally sensitive way. The resource suggests that black and ethnic minority people should be involved in patient simulation exercises, and that GPs in training should be in contact with ethnic minority communities. The resource is intended for GP registrars and medical students but also useful for other professionals, and would be very valuable for doctors in palliative medicine. Kai observes, "Overlooking them, and thus failing to address our own awareness and attitudes may explain why important initiatives such as ethnic monitoring have faltered" (1999 172). Questions of open surgery rather than appointment systems needed to be discussed with ethnic minority communities in their relevant languages. A valuable suggestion from the RCGP resource was that inner-city GPs should be involved in curriculum development for GPs in training, and that the latter should have placements in multicultural practices (Yee 1997). It was beyond the scope of this document to find out from medical schools how far this resource has been implemented, or about the programmes of education about ethnic minorities already in place, although Bower and Patel (1998) refer to bid by the Department of General practice at the University of Birmingham and Birmingham Health Authority "to ensure that issues around black and minority ethnic communities were integrated throughout undergraduate medical training. This was one of only five bids funded across the country" (Bower and Patel 1998).

However, the issue is not just one of culturally sensitive care, but care for the *dying* and their families. Medical professionals often have difficulty facing their own emotions about death, let alone those of their patients (Katz 2000, Buckman 2001). As Buckman points out, medical training tends to encourage the view that when a patient deteriorates it is someone's fault – "there is little or no teaching on the subject of what to do when the disease cannot be reversed" (p.151). Many doctors are not trained to deal with emotional reactions and feel uncomfortable with them, particularly if they do not know how to deal with their own feelings. Admitting they do not know the answer is often very difficult. Buckman also refers to 'counter-phobic behaviour' in which the professionals who are actually afraid of mortality deny this by becoming a doctor, to reinforce a sense of their own invulnerability. An unfamiliar culture might complicate the way in which issues of disclosure are dealt with, particularly if there are stereotypical perceptions and fears of 'emotional outbursts'.

Until there is a profound shift from an ethnocentric biomedical perspective to a multicultural or pluralist one, ethnic minority patients will be seen as 'other', and a problem, rather than welcomed as an opportunity and challenge. This means embedding a broad interdisciplinary multicultural education early into medical and nursing education, with a thoroughgoing anti-discrimination component, and an understanding of sociology. The development of cultural competence is relevant to all healthcare professionals in a multicultural context. The advantage of this would not just be for ethnic minority patients, but for all patients who too often are seen in terms of a disease rather than people who have their own perspectives, health beliefs, and anxieties about care. Kai observes:

> In the wider context, primary care for many patients from ethnic minorities reflects the general demands of care for all socioeconomically disadvantaged communities. PCTs need targeted support and resources in these circumstances. The imminent retirement of a cohort of doctors from minority ethnic backgrounds who have sustained general practice in many inner-city areas adds greater urgency. PCG-led decision-making now offers important opportunities to begin addressing these issues and to advance service development that is responsive to local communities' needs… If we can learn to value this diversity then we will bring mutual benefits for our patients and ourselves (Kai 1999:172).

10.5. Nursing education

The knowledge and skills referred to above cannot be contained in 'fact-files' but demand quite long and intensive training. This has to go beyond the half-day or so on multi-cultural aspects of death and dying that is often included in post-graduate palliative care courses. The statutory bodies acknowledge the need to provide curricula which will enable nurses to develop appropriate holistic care for ethnic minorities,[2] which needs to be translated into "practice and the processes they need to engage in to develop skills to deliver ethnically sensitive care" (Gerrish 1997:361). This requires a commitment at all levels to incorporate it into nursing education. Gerrish *et al.*, in a survey of training institutions, found that only a few were committed to providing an appropriate curriculum with cultural competencies, although there were examples of good practice. Many, however, provided no more than a token response or felt that such training was irrelevant because the institution was not located in an area with a big ethnic minority population. Since Trusts were likely to assess the necessity of such training on the basis of the demographic distribution of their populations, they may well not prioritise transcultural training in nursing education:

> Consequently, there is a need for professional and statutory bodies to take a lead in making this a national rather than a local issue. This is perhaps critically so, given the unambiguous evidence from current teachers and mentors that many do not feel competent in being able to teach transcultural competencies. The lack of transcultural competence and confidence within the current nursing professions indicates the need for a systematic provision of post-regis-tration continuing education. (Gerrish et al, 1996:102-103)

The question of what such training should involve raises some of the issues already referred to above. Culley (1996) states that it is not adequate to provide a "curricular dose of 'other cultures'", arguing instead for "The inclusion of social scientific concepts and analyses into the nurse education curriculum [to provide] an opportunity to discuss the more complex ways in which social relations and social structures impact upon minorities." (1996:569). She does not, however, include suggestions for ways in which such a training can move beyond the

---

2 UKCC 1989. UKCC requirements for the content of Project 2000
programmes. PS&D/89/04(B), UKCC; London, National Health Service and
Community Care Act 1990; English National Board 1989, *Standard, Kind and
Content of Project 2000 Courses*, ENB, London.

political and socio-economic debate at an intellectual level, to provide a practical reality for nurse who have to engage daily with ethnic minority patients.

Gerrish (1997) takes up the issue with a broader remit. Nurses are trained to provide care within the dominant majority's cultural value system, and are not working within a culture free, but a culturally determined framework, so the challenge is to provide training that incorporates self awareness as well as cultural sensitivity. Citing Lynam (1992), she makes four recommendations:

- There has to be a balance between introducing ethno-specific knowledge and cross-cultural approaches. Lynam warns against overloading cultural information about any specific group as this can lead to stereotyping.
- Nurses have to have the skills to utilise this knowledge in the context of the patient-nurse relationship, so that it is a partnership in learning.
- They also need to have a critical understanding of the wider context of the political and socio-economic influences which influence the healthcare systems and cultural bias.
- Students have to be aware of and sensitive to their own culture, attitudes, and values, as well as the cultural milieu of the nursing environment. This includes being willing to recognise and challenge the dominance of the prevailing bio-medical models of health and a recognition of the validity of other models.

These concepts can be incorporated into the curriculum by various strategies such as experiential workshops, exercises designed to help the students examine their own cultural preconceptions, video-recordings of interactions between nurses and patients, and ethnographic research projects. Encouraging self-examination and reflection while working in a multicultural context and actively engaging in participant observation in such a context are also suggested. Exercises and case studies are also provided by Papadopoulis *et al.* (1998), to be used for personal reflection, analysis and role-play.

No amount of exercise in a classroom will be effective without contact with members of ethnic minority communities. The concepts of cultural competence and safety are clearly relevant in this context, as well as the recognition that working in a transcultural context involves emotional work and the development of empathy through referential grounding (Gunaratnam *et al.* 1998, cf. 11.3 above). While such policies have been found to be been successful with students and teachers, Gerrish points out that the effect on patient outcomes has not been evaluated in a systematic way, so this is an area for future research.

10.6. Recruiting ethnic minority nurses

The need to recruit more black and Asian health professionals into palliative care services was highlighted by Hill and Penso. It is difficult to ascertain the numbers of ethnic minority nurses (and doctors) in palliative care (Gunaratnam, personal communication). Shortage of ethnic minority staff in palliative care and in management continues to be a problem (Pitches 2000, Tanzeem Ahmed 1998). According to Gerrish *et al.* (1996), the relative proportion of ethnic minority nurses to the population at large is high, (approximately 8% compared with 6% from the general population). Of these figures, twice as many identify themselves as Black (including Black African and Black Caribbean) as S. Asian, although Sadler (1999) suggests that as the older generation of West Indian nurses retire they are not being replaced. The reasons for lower Asian figures have been attributed to cultural factors, such as negative attitudes to the nursing profession, especially for marriageable women, and the desire of parents for their children to enter more prestigious professions such as medicine (Karseras and Hopkins 1987, Cassidy 1995). Gerrish *et al.* (1996) argue this is not borne out by all the literature. A research and development project by Bradford and Airedale Health Related Strategy Group to find out why the recruitment of Asian nurses was low found that students were put off by a "'bedpan' image of nursing, seeing it as 'physically demanding' but 'mentally unstimulating'" (Sadler 1999:14). Some felt it would be culturally unacceptable to nurse male patients in bed, and there was concern about the appropriateness of nursing uniforms. Other factors such as poor perceptions of nursing as a career because of television programmes like *Casualty* (Bharj 1995), the perceived low status of the profession, institutional racism, and negative experiences of the NHS are all possibilities. In 1995 a Policy Studies Institute survey found that "two-thirds of black and Asian nurses had reported racist harassment from patients and from their white colleagues" (The Parekh report 2000:191). The problem of recruitment is also an issue for Greek Cypriots, because while they wish to be cared for by members of their own community, they are reluctant to allow their children to enter the nursing profession (Papadopoulos 1998).

As ethnic monitoring on recruitment is still inadequate it is difficult to judge how successful recruitment strategies are. However, Gerrish (1997) suggests that the English Nursing Board data indicate that even those from ethnic minorities who do apply to train are less likely to get places on nursing courses. Recruitment into nursing *per se,* and into palliative care nursing, are two different issues, and it may be the case that special strategies are needed to attract experienced ethnic minority nurses into palliative care. It is important that ethnic minority individuals who do come into the palliative care services should not, as Somerville (2001) comments, be used as an alternative to good advocacy schemes, or be treated as the 'experts' on their particular 'culture', which may be far removed from that of the patients and their families. To use them as interpreters and advocates abuses their training and prevents them from getting on with their work. Gerrish *et al.* (1996) see ethnic minority staff as a valuable resource in professional education and training as well, but also acknowledges that they can be exploited and abused, and used as a "panacea for the majority professional's failure to take responsibility for their acquisition of transcultural skills as teachers and practitioners." (p.1996:103)

Chapter 11

Conclusion and recommendations

There is clearly a commitment to improve access to palliative care for members of ethnic minority groups. The first stage should be a determined programme of stocktaking to see how far Hill and Penso's recommendations have been followed. This needs to be extended to a comprehensive audit using different auditing systems. Ahmedzai stresses the importance of fulfilling special needs and ensuring the audit systems are good enough to pick this up (personal communication). It is evident that a great deal of work still needs to be done to ascertain what their needs and requirements are, and whether supply matches these. Information about ethnic minority needs is required at several levels. Information about epidemiology and morbidity and mortality rates have to be accurate. Because cancer is not the predominant cause of illness and death in many ethnic minority groups, there are also issues about the provision of palliative care to specific diseases, or whether it should be available to all. Most of the epidemiological information so far is based on 1991 Census statistics, and the latest accurate data will not be available for another year or so (Bhopal and Balarajan, personal communication). Accurate HES data should be forthcoming but as Aspinall shows, is not yet being collected correctly. Without ethnic monitoring it is not possible to tell whether the supply of services is adequate, and whether there is an uptake commensurate with need.

At a second level, there has to be further information about local communities from both demographic and sociological perspectives, their attitudes to palliative care services as well as their requirements and whether or not the available services actually meet local needs. Such issues include where death should take place, who should care for the dying and whether in fact they can or will do so. At a third level, more information is needed about religious, spiritual and cultural care requirements, taking into account both individual and community perceptions of health and disease. To obtain all this information requires in-depth ethnographic studies of different communities, prospective studies of patients and carers and retrospective studies of carers. There are still too many gaps, with little or no information about the palliative care needs of smaller communities such as the diverse African groups (including refugee groups such as Somalis) and 'white' minorities.

A major factor in improving access is better outreach through the involvement of ethnic minorities in decision making, and planning, first through discussion and negotiation with individuals, then with community organisations and focus groups. This is already being undertaken, as has been noted, in a number of on-going projects and established services such as the Acorn Children's Hospice (Notta and Warr), The North London Hospice (Oliviere), St.Catherine's Hospice (Simmonds and Mount), in Birmingham (Pitches), and Warwickshire (Webb and Young). Their expertise and insights need to be shared. The involvement needs to be at all levels. Simmonds (2001), with reference to Crawley, comments:

> South Asian community and religious leaders all agreed that things are changing rapidly in the Asian communities as successive generations embrace western patterns of education and employment, which will make traditional approaches to caring difficult to achieve. At a focus group for Asian community and religious leaders a future need for palliative care was very much recognised. It was suggested, both during the interview and focus group phase, that someone from the Asian communities should be appointed to the Board of Trustees. These participants stressed the importance of representation for ethnic minority communities starting from the top of the management structure of the Hospice. At ground level, it was suggested that an ethnic minority liaison worker could be appointed to help medical staff provide a culturally sensitive service and to create and maintain strong links with the Asian communities.

Involving community leaders is important but not sufficient because of local politics – individual leaders may change as temple, church, mosque or gurdwara committees change (cf. Firth 1997). Links with both formal and informal groups by bi-lingual ethnic minority nurses and/or linkworkers, as well as active informal engagement by other staff with communities will have a positive effect on both sides. Attendance by primary and palliative care health workers at festivals, functions, and especially, funerals and paying condolence visits are all forms of outreach which have a remarkable effect on communities which may be feeling marginalised. Gunaratnam (2001c) stresses the need to see cultural differences in *relational* terms between the cultural identity of the organisation and the service user, and not just in terms of the user, who thus becomes an

'Other'. Equity of care does not necessary mean the same care, but individualised care according to need. The concept of supportive care as a complement to palliative care seems to provide a way ahead that involves partnership at all levels, provided it expands to include concepts of cultural competence, and engages the family and community as well as the individual patient.

11.1. Recommendations

The following recommendations make both general and research suggestions arising from the preceding chapters that relate to specialist palliative care services. Some of the recommendations are based on the original recommendations in *Opening Doors*, which are still pertinent.

1. Review of the practical consequences of *Opening Doors*

- An exercise should be undertaken to examine how far the recommendations of *Opening Doors* (1995) have actually been put into practice in different PC organisations throughout England and Wales.
- The above exercise needs to be extended to a comprehensive audit using different auditing systems, which have to be good enough to pick special needs of ethnic minority patients. A published standard such as the Kings Fund Hospital Quality system, covering issues such as privacy and appropriate food could be used as an audit measure.

2. Access and provision

- Areas of good practice need highlighting and the experience and recommendations made available within the service. In particular, it would be useful to note where there are excellent advocacy/linkworker services and the role and training of these workers, the education of staff, links with the local community, and culturally sensitive services.
- There need to be national standards for monitoring factors relating to disadvantage, poverty and racism, which affect health and adequate access to care, in order to determine need and demand.
- The question of whether palliative care should be offered to all terminally ill patients, regardless of whether they have cancer or not, needs to be addressed.

- Community involvement with Hospice and Specialist Palliative Care Services needs to be expanded so that ethnic minority users have input into their own needs, requirements and care. Members of ethnic minority communities should be represented on management committees at all levels.
- National standards need to be established, with nationally validated qualifications for the training of advocates, linkworkers and interpreters, with specialist training in palliative care and the breaking of bad news.

3. Cultural sensitivity

- There needs to be a continuous examination of the language used to describe 'black and ethnic minorities', preferably in favour of 'diversity', 'pluralism' and 'multi-culturalism', to avoid stereotyping, pathologising them, creating victims or turning them into 'others'.
- Contact should be maintained with local ethnic minority communities and their places of worship and organisations. Voluntary organisations should be encouraged to participate with appropriate support and bereavement visiting.
- Each unit should have appropriate resources with information, nursing aids such as pain charts, dictionaries and phrase books for use in the absence of adequate interpreters.
- Notices in appropriate languages, name labels or badges for identification of staff, and multifaith chapels contribute to a more user-friendly atmosphere.
- There should be written information about names in different languages, religious and cultural traditions, and correct forms of address, along with the accepted forms of greetings.

4. Ethnic monitoring

- Accurate ethnic monitoring of PC services needs to be strongly reinforced, with a broader breakdown of ethnic and religious categories to include different 'white' groups such as Greeks, Turks, Welsh and Irish, and different religions.
- Monitoring and HES should be accurate and give as much detail about the patient's self-assigned ethnicity as possible.

5. Care issues

■ Hospitals and hospices need to provide culturally sensitive palliative care with adequate interpreting/advocacy services, a culturally sensitive disclosure policy, and adequate discharge policies. This involves on-going in-service training in anti-discrimination as well as cultural competence.

■ Dietary and religious requirements should be discussed fully with users on an individual basis, so that there is provision for special needs, including water for ablutions, prayer time/space, skin, hair and hygiene needs, and appropriate clothing or gowns for patients.

■ Ethnic minority staff should be recruited where possible, and advocates/interpreters made readily available.

■ Ensure that if home care is the preferred option, the financial and support needs of carers are taken into account, allowing for sensitive handling of the position of informal carers vis a vis their own communities. This has resource implications.

■ Appropriate Day Care has to ensure dietary needs are met on an individual basis, that there are carers and/or interpreters speaking the appropriate languages and both emotional and practical support can be offered.

■ Anti-racism and anti-discrimination policies have to be firmly established and met at all levels of care, including protection from racist patients.

■ Community support should not be taken for granted and the involvement of children in caring needs to be monitored.

■ The significance of the family in many communities has to be recognised as a matter of policy, and appropriate provision made for large numbers to visit dying inpatients in separate rooms.

6. Religion and spirituality

■ Palliative care staff need to be educated about religion and spirituality in different faiths, since they affect disclosure issues, beliefs about care and the manner and place of death, attitudes to pain control, and bereavement.

■ Training in spiritual care has to include a multi-faith dimension, which is able to see beyond a view of religion as mainly to do with rituals and belief, to a search for meaning and the recognition of the transcendent for members of religious faiths.

■ Access to priests, imams, ministers, granthis or other functionaries has to be ensured. Chaplains can play an important role in enabling dialogue and sharing to take place.

- There has to be sensitivity to the use of Christian symbols in settings with people of other faiths, especially Muslims and Jews.

7. Medical professionals

- In order to ensure appropriate referrals to specialist palliative care services, there needs to be an organised system of information provision for hospital consultants and GPs about available palliative care services for ethnic minority patients. This could be done through the National Council for Hospice and Specialist Palliative Care Services and the relevant Health Sector organisations in each area, the BMA and journal articles.
- At a local level there should be a regular programme of meetings with community leaders, patient representatives and focus groups, to enable medical professionals to develop an understanding and awareness of local communities and the context of their patients' lives, health beliefs and behaviours and attitude to death.
- GPs and consultants need to ensure adequate interpreting and advocacy services, and ensure that their receptionists understand the needs of patients and can access local services rapidly if they are not already in place.
- The recommendations by the RCGP should be incorporated into under- and post-graduate training, especially for those in general practice and palliative medicine. A broad interdisciplinary multicultural component into medical training which includes some grounding in medical sociology with regard to health beliefs and explanatory systems would help guard against an ethnocentric biomedical perspective.
- GP managed palliative care teams may need to be adapted to ethnic minority needs to provide culturally sensitive care.
- Appropriate literature about palliative care and ethnic minorities needs to be written for medical and nursing training.

8. Nursing training and recruitment

- Training in culturally competent nursing should begin at undergraduate level and continue as in-service programmes rather than be provided in short 'cultural doses'.
- A policy of culturally competent care needs to be in place in each organisation which would allow on-going opportunities to share anxieties and experiences, continuous development and opportunities to engage with ethnic minority communities outside the practice.

- Recruitment of nurses from different ethnic communities for palliative care should be made a priority. Apprehensions about dealing with dying patients could be overcome by recruiting experienced nurses.
- Communities, such as the Bangladeshis, should be encouraged to allow their young women to train, to ensure a pool of nurses who could serve those communities in the future.
- Ethnic minority volunteers should be recruited to provide help and support in Day Centres and inpatient care.

9. Anti-racism, anti-discrimination and equal opportunities

- There needs to be a code of conduct incorporating an anti-discriminatory and anti-racist philosophy for health professionals as well as patients.
- There has to be a clearly defined equal opportunities strategy in place, adopted by purchasers and providers, as well as a programme of implementation with measures to monitor quality and assess change.

10. Bereavement support

- Proper bereavement support training needs to be established for ethnic minority individuals, recruiting, whenever possible, local members of the different communities. Majority community individuals offering support also need appropriate training.
- A training manual, which can be readily obtainable nationally and adapted to local use, should be commissioned.

11. Information provision

- Available information about palliative care services in different languages needs to be pooled and made available at a national level. A national database could be produced on the Web, which could be readily accessed and adapted to local requirements.
- The use of well-trained bi-lingual support workers, advocates and linkworkers are also important sources of information for the communities and for the health professionals.

11.2. Research suggestions

1. Beliefs and attitudes to illness and death

- There needs to be more research into the health beliefs and explanatory systems of ethnic minority groups in the UK, particularly with reference to stigmatising diseases such as HIV/AIDS and cancer, which may contribute to late presentation for diagnosis and treatment.

- Related to the above, research is needed into attitudes to alternative (especially folk and traditional) medicine and western medicine in terms of health beliefs and traditions. This would throw light on issues of compliance with medication and treatment.

- The language of distress and illness behaviour in different ethnic minority groups needs further research to enable appropriate palliative care to be offered.

- In-depth ethnographic research needs to be undertaken into beliefs and attitudes about death and bereavement in a wide range of communities, perhaps in cooperation with university departments of anthropology, medical sociology, and South Asian and ethnic studies.

2. Care

- Further research is needed into the roles of carers in Hindu and Muslim groups not already researched, and smaller groups such as the Chinese, Turks and Greeks.

- Care preferences for users needs to be established by a number of short-term research projects in different geographic areas.

- The palliative care needs of different refugee groups needs researching, bearing in mind their special difficulties.

- Further research into the needs and attitudes of ethnic minority women, both as patients and carers, would make it easier to provide appropriate and sensitive care and support.

- Research is needed into the problems of ageing in those communities not so far studied, especially 'white' minorities such as the Jewish community and the Irish community to ascertain possible palliative care needs and demands in the future, and to ascertain the kind of care that is already potentially available.

- Palliative care provision for ethnic minority people in hospital needs to be researched in different hospital trusts, including adequate monitoring, interpreting or advocacy services, discharge policies and a study of what actually happens at discharge. Shortfalls of provision and care need to be ascertained and remedied. This is related to 11.1, question 1, but would focus on in-patient hospital care.
- Access to and provision of specialist palliative care services in terms of local demography needs to be researched by each health authority, in liaison with the local communities.
- The numbers of dying patients and bodies returned to their homeland needs to be researched to give some idea of the numbers, and indicate to what extent they affect the mortality statistics.

3. Disclosure, autonomy and informed consent
- Research is needed into different religious/cultural communities on attitudes to disclosure, informed consent and patient autonomy and whether these are shared equally by patients and relatives.

4. Pain
- Comparative studies on attitudes and responses to pain in different communities in the UK would enhance understanding of approaches to pain relief and withdrawal of treatment.

5. Referrals
- Research needs to be done into GP referrals in different areas. In particular, the attitudes and referral patterns of ethnic minority doctors would provide more information into their attitudes to the local ethnic minority communities, levels of 'gatekeeping', and the extent to which they are familiar with palliative care services.

Bibliography on Ethnic Minorities and Palliative Care

Acheson, D, 1998, *Independent Inquiry Into Inequalities in Health: Report,* London: The Stationery Office.

Acheson, K D, 1999, 'Equality of Health: dream or reality?' *Journal of the Royal College of Physicians,* 33. (1): 70-77.

Ades, A E, J Walker, B Bolling, D Cubitt, R Jones, 1999, 'The effect of the world-wide epidemic of HIV prevalence in the UK': record linkage in anonymous seroprevalence surveys', *AIDS,* Dec 3, 13 (17), 2437-2443.

Addington-Hall, Julia, and Dan Altman, 2000, 'Which terminally ill cancer patients in the United Kingdom receive care from community specialist palliative care nurses?' *Journal of Advanced Nursing,* 32(4), 799-806.

Addington-Hall, Julia, Dan Altman and J M McCarthy, 1998, 'Which terminally ill cancer patients receive hospice in-patient care?' *Social Science and Medicine,* 1998:46:1011-1016.

Addington-Hall, Julia, and J M McCarthy, 1995, 'Regional study of care for the dying: methods and sample characteristics', *Palliative Medicine,* 9, 27-35.

Addington-Hall, Julia, P West, S Karlsen and M West, 1999, 'Care in the Last Years of Life in Lambeth, Southwark and Lewisham: final report', Department of Palliative Care and Policy, Kings College, London.

Age Concern: 2000, *Age and Race: Double Discrimination: Life in Britain.*

Ahmed, S, 1999, 'Coronary heart disease: the Indian Asian diet', *Nursing Standard,* March 224, Vol13(27).

Ahmed, Tanzeem, 1998, 'The Asian experience' in Rawaf, Salman and Veena Bahl (eds), pp319-328.

Ahmad, W, (ed), 1993, *Race and Health in Contemporary Britain,* Buckingham, Open University Press.

— 1996 'Family obligations and social change among Asian communities', in Ahmed, W and K Atkin, pp51-72.

Ahmad, W, and Karl Atkin (eds), 1996, *'Race' and Community Care,* Buckingham, Open University Press.

Ahmad, W, E Kernohan and M Baker, 1989, 'Patients' choice of general practitioner: influence of patients' fluency in English and the ethnicity and sex of the doctor', *Journal of the Royal College of General Practitioners,* Vol 39, pp153-155

Ahmad, Waqar, Trevor Sheldon, Ossie Stuart *et al.,* 1996, *Ethnicity and Health: Reviews of Literature and Guidance for Purchasers in the Areas of Cardiovascular Disease, Mental Health and Haemoglobinopathies,* Social Policy Research Unit and the NHS Centre for Reviews and Dissemination.

Ahmedzai, S, 2000, 'The Sheffield model of Suportive Care', *The Sheffield Palliative Care Studies Group Annual Review,* June 2000.

Ahmedzai, Sam H and Declan Walsh, 2000, 'Palliative medicine and modern cancer care', *Seminars in Oncology*, Vol 27, No 1, 1-6.

Albury, David, Andrena Cumella, Jeff Rodrigues and Rukshana Kapasi, nd. *Beyond the Boundary: an Action Guide for Health Service Purchasers-Consultation and Involvement,* Office for Public management and NHS Ethnic Health Unit.

Aldous J, M Bardsley, R Daniell, R Gair, B Jacobson, C Lowdell, D Morgan, M Storkey and G Taylor, 1999, *Refugee Health in London.* London: The Health of Londoners Project.

Alexander, Ziggi, 1999, *Study of Black, Asian and Ethnic Minority Issues,* Department of Health.

Alibhai-Brown, 'Age of Respect: The Way Society Treats Older People from Ethnic Minorities', *Community Care,* 10-16 Dec 1998, pp24-25

Allan, Simon, 1999, 'Palliative care in New Zealand', Letter to Editor, *Progress in Palliative Care* 7(3)1999 120-121.

A Matter of Chance for Carers: the report of the national inspection of local authority support for carers, DOH/SSI.

Andrews, Margaret M and Joyceen S Boyle, *Transcultural Concepts in Nursing Care*, Philadelphia, Lipincott Williams and Wilkins.

Anionwu, E, 'Welcoming Ethnic Diversity within Nursing and Midwifery Education', *NT Research*, Vol 3, No 5, 1998, pp361-363.

Archibald, Graeme, 2000, 'The needs of South Asians with a terminal illness', *Professional Nurse,* Feb 2000, 15.5, 316-319.

Aspinall, Peter J, 1998, 'Describing the 'white' ethnic group and its composition in medical research', *Soc.Sci. Med*, Vol 47 No 11 pp 1797-1808

— 1999a, 'Ethnic groups and Our Healthier Nation: Whither the information age?' *Journal of Public Health Medicine*, Vol 21, No 2, pp125-132.

— 1999b, Letter: 'Mental health and Irish ethnicity' in *British Journal of Psychiatry,* 1999, 175:92.

— 2000a, 'The challenges of measuring the ethno-cultural diversity of Britain in the new millennium', *Policy & Politics*, Vol 28, No 1, 109-118.

— 2000b, 'The mandatory collection of data on ethnic group of inpatients: experience of NHS trusts in England in the first reporting years', *Public Health*, 114l, 254-259.

— 2000c, Reply to Koffman and Higginson in '*Journal of Public Health Medicine*', Vol 22, No 2, pp246.

Association of London Government, 2000, *Sick of Being Excluded.* London: ALG.

Atkin, Karl, Waqar I U Ahmad and Elizabeth Anionwu, 1998, "Screening and counselling for sickle cell disorders and thalassaemia: the experience of parents and health professionals', *Soc. Sci. Med.* Vol 47, 11, 1639-1651.

Atkin, K, E Cameron, F Badger and H Evers, 'Asian Elders' Knowledge and Future Use of Community Social and Health Services', *New Community,* 15(3), April 1989 pp439-449

Atkin, K, and Rollings, J, 1996, 'Looking after their own? Family care-giving among Asian and Afro-Caribbean communities', in Ahmad, W and K Atkin, pp73-86.

Atri, J, M Falshaw, A Livingstone, J Robson, for Healthy Eastenders Project, 1996, 'Fair shares in health care? Ethnic and socio-economic influences on recording of preventive care in selected inner London general practices', *BMJ* Vol 312, March 6, pp 614-617.

Bahl, Veena, 1996a, 'Cancer and ethnic minorities – the Department of Health's perspective', *British Journal of Cancer*, 1996, 74, Supp XXIX, S2-S10.

— 1996b, *Directory of Ethnic Minority Initiatives*, May 1996, Department of Health.

Balarajan, Rasaratnam, 1996, 'Ethnicity and variations in the nation's health', *Health Trends*, 27:4:114-119.

Balarajan, R, and V Soni Raleigh, 1995, *Ethnicity and Health in England*, NHS, Ethnic Health Unit, London, HMSO.

Ballard, P, I Finlay, N Jones, C Searle, S Roberts, 1998, 'Spiritual Perspectives among terminally ill patients: a Welsh Sample', *Modern Believing*, Vol 41.2. pp30-38.

Ballard, R, 2000, 'Culture, Race and Ethnicity: A definitional perspective', University of Manchester, unpublished document.

Bardsley, Martin, John Hamm, Caroline Lowdell, David Morgan and Marian Storkey, 2000, *Developing Health Assessment for Black and Minority Ethnic Groups: Analysing Routine Health Information*, Health of Londoners Project.

Bardsley, Martin and Caroline Lowdell, 1999, *Health Monitoring for Black and Minority Ethnic Groups*, produced for the London Health Strategy, Health of Londoners Project.

Barot, Rohit, (1993), *Religion and Ethnicity: Minorities and Social change in the Metropolis*, Kampen, Kok Pharos Publishing House.

Barot, Rohit, Harriet Bradley and Steve Fenton, 1999, *Ethnicity Gender and Social Change*, Basingstoke, Macmillan Press Ltd.

Barry, C, 'Croydon Home Care Ethnicity project, abstract', *Palliative Medicine*, 1998, Vol 12, No 6, pp 493-494.

Bates, Maryann S, 1987, 'Ethnicity and pain: a biocultural model', *Soc. Sci. Med.* 24:1: 47-50

Baxter, Carol, Akgul Baylav, Jon Fuller, Alan Marr, Marsha Sanders, 1996, 'The Case for the Provision of Bilingual Services within the NHS', *Bilingual Health Advocacy Project,* Lawsson Practice, St. Leonard's Hospital, funded by the Department of Health

Baxter, M S, 1987, 'Ethnicity and pain: a biocultural model', *Social Science and Medicine*, 24.1.

Becker, Robert, 1999, 'Teaching communication with the dying across cultural boundaries', *British Journal of Nursing*, 8 (14): 938-942.

Beishon, S, s Virdee and A Hagell, 1995, *Nursing in a Multi-Ethnic NHS,* London: Policy Studies Institute.

Beliappa, J, 1991, *Illness or Distress? Alternative models of mental health,* London, Confederation of Indian Organisations.

Bell, Truda S, Lucy K Branston, Robert Newcombe and Garry Barton, 'Interventions to improve uptake of breast screening in inner-city Cardiff general practices with ethnic minority lists', *Ethnicity and Health*, 1999, 4(4) 277-284

Berkovits, Dayan B, 1992, *Guide to Jewish Practice for Nurses and Medical Staff,* 2nd (revised) edition (selection).

Beyond the Boundary: An Action Guide for Health Service Purchasers – Consultation and Involvement. nd, Health Care for Black and Minority Ethnic People, NHS Ethnic Health Unit, Leeds.

Bhakta, Padma, Peter Donnelly and John Mayberry, 1995, 'management of breast disease in Asian women, *Professional Nurse*, Dec 1995, 11 (3):187-189.

Bharj, K K, 1995, *Nurse recruitment: an Asian Response,* Race Relations Research Unit, University of Bradford and Bradford and Ilkley Community College.

Bhopal, Raj, 1997, 'Is research into ethnicity and health racist, unsound or important science?' *BMJ,* 314, June 14, 1751-1758.

— 1998, 'Spectre of racism in health and health care: lessons from history and the United States', *BMJ* 316, 1970-1973.

Bhopal, Raj and Liam Donaldson, 1998, 'White, European, Western, Caucasian, or what? Inappropriate labelling in research on race, ethnicity, and health', *American Journal of Public Health*, Sept 1998, 88 (9):103-7.

Black, D, 1999, 'A Black look at the independent inquiry into inequalities in Health', *Journal of the Royal College of Physicians,* Vol 33 No 2, Mar/April 1999:148-149.

Blakemore, Ken, 2000, 'Health and social care needs in minority communities: an over-problemetized issue?' *Health and Social Care in the Community,* 8(1) 22-30.

Bodell, Janet and Marie-Ange Weng, 2000, 'The Jewish patient and terminal dehydration: a hospice ethical dilemma', *American Journal of Hospice and Palliative Care,* 17 (3) May/June.

Boneham, M, K E Williams, J R M Copeland, P McKibbin, K Wilson, A Scott, and P A Saunders, 1997, 'Elderly people from ethnic minorities: mental illness, unmet need and barriers to service use', *Health and Social Care in the Community*, 5(3), 173-180.

Bower, Cynthia and Moosa Patel, 1998, *Action Plan for Black and Minority Ethnic Communities,* Birmingham Health Authority, Nov 1998, Directorate of Primary Care Development.

Bowes, A M, and T M Domokos, 1995, 'Key issues in South Asian women's health: a study in Glasgow', *Social Sciences in Health,* 1(3):145-157.

Bowling, A, M Farquhar and J Leaver, 1992, 'Jewish People and ageing: their emotional well-being, physical health status and use of services, *Nurse Practitioner,* 5 (4):5-6.

Bradshaw, Ann, 1997, 'Teaching spiritual care to nurses; an alternative approach', *International Journal of Palliative Care,* Vol 3, No 1, Jan-Feb, 51-57.

Bremner, Isobel, *Improving Access to Hospice Services by Black and Ethnic Minority Communities*, St. Christopher's Hospice, nd.

Brenner, Paul R, 1997, 'Issues of Access in a Diverse Society', *Hospice Journal,* 1997:12:2:9-16.

Brent & Harrow Health Agency *et al.,* 1995, *Brent & Harrow Refugee Survey.* London: Brent & Harrow Health Agency, Brent & Harrow Refugee Groups, Northwest London Training and Enterprise Council,

Brooks, N, P Magee, G Bhatti, C Briggs, S Buckley, S Guthrie, H Moltesen, C Moore, S Murray, 2000, 'Asian patients' perspective on the communication facilities provided in a large inner city hospital', *Journal of Clinical Nursing,* 2000: 9: 706-712.

Buckman, Robert, 2001, 'Communication in palliative care: a practical guide', in Dickenson, Donna, Malcolm Johnson and Jeanne Katz, pp146-173.

Burghart, Richard (ed), 1987, *Hinduism in Great Britain: the Perpetuation of Religion in an Alien Cultural Milieu*, London, Tavistock.

Callan, Alyson and Roland Littlewood, 1998, 'Patient satisfaction: ethnic origin or explanatory model?' *International Journal of Social Psychiatry,* 1998 44(1) 1-11.

Calman, Kenneth C, 1997, 'Equity, poverty and health for all', *BMJ,* Vol 314, 19 April, 1997, 1187-91.

Calman, Kenneth and Deidre Hine, 1995, *A Policy Framework for commissioning cancer services: a Report by the expert advisory group on cancer to the chief medical officers of England a Wales. Guidance for purchasers and providers of cancer services.*

Cancer Research Campaign, 'Cancer and Minority Ethnic Groups', *British Journal of Cancer,* Vol 74, Sept 1996

Cassidy J, 1995, 'Ethnic dilemmas', *Nursing Times,* 91,18.

Chambers, Jacky, 2000, *Health Improvement Programme Position Statement,* Director of Public Health, Birmingham HA, Birmingham

Champion, T, Population Review: (3) Migration to, from and within the UK. *Population Trends,* 1996, Spring (83): 5-16.

Chan, Christine, 2000, 'The quality of life of women of Chinese origin', *Health and Social Care in the Community,* 8(3), 212-222

Chan, Joanne Y K, 1995, 'Dietary beliefs of Chinese patients', *Nursing Standard,* March 29, Vol 9 No 27, 30-35.

Chandra, Jeff, 1996, *Facing up to difference: a toolkit for creating culturally competent health services for Black and Minority Ethnic communities,* London: Kings Fund.

Chandra, Jeff, Josam Associates, 1996, *A Culture of Quality: Guidelines for Monitoring Health Service Performance on Ethnic Health,* A report prepared for the NHS Ethnic Health Unit, Leeds.

Chaturvedi, Harbinder Rai, Yoav Ben-Schlomo, 1997, 'Lay diagnosis and health-care-seeking behaviour for chest pain in South Asians and Europeans', *The Lancet,* 1997, 350:1578-83.

Chung, Ki Tak, Peter French and Sylvia Chan, 1999, 'Patient-related barriers to cancer pain management in a Palliative Care setting', *Cancer Nursing* 1999, 22 (3):196-203.

Chung, Young, 2000, 'Palliative care in Korea: a nursing point of view', *Progress in Palliative Care,* 8, (1):2000.

Clarke, Colin, Ceri Peach and Steven Vertovec (eds.), 1990, *South Asians Overseas: Migration and Ethnicity,* Cambridge, Cambridge University Press.

Cleeland, C S, R Govin, L Baez, P Loehrer, K J Padya, 'Pain and Treatment of Pain in minority patients with cancer', *Annals of Internal Medicine,* 1997, Nov 1:127 (9): 813-6.

Cliffe, S, *et al.,* 1999, 'Surveillance for the impact in the UK of HIV epidemics in S. Asia', *Ethnicity and Health, 1999,* Feb-Mar; 4 (1-2): 5 18.

Cobb, Mark and Vanessa Robshaw (eds) 1998, *The Spiritual Challenge of Health Care,* Edinburgh, Churchill and Livingstone.

Cole, Owen, and Piara Singh Sambhi, 1978, *The Sikhs: Their Religious Beliefs and Practices,* London, Routledge and Kegan Paul

Cooke, M, S Wilson, P Cox, A Roalfe, 2000, 'Public understanding of medical terminology: non-English speakers may not receive optimal care', *Journal of Accid. Emerg. Med.,* 2000: 17:119-121.

Coup, Anne, 1996, 'Cultural Safety and culturally congruent care: a comparative analysis of Irhapeti Ramsden's and Madeleine Leininger's educational projects for practice', *Nursing Praxis in New Zealand,* March 1996, Vol 11, No 1 4-11.

Cowles, Cathleen V, 1996, 'Cultural Perspectives of grief: an expanded concept analysis', *Journal of Advanced Nursing* 1996, 23, 187-194

Cortis, Joseph Domenic, 2000, 'Perceptions and Experiences with Nursing Care: a study of Pakistani (Urdu) communities in the UK', *Journal of Transcultural Nursing,* Vol 11, No 2, April 2000, 111-118.

Currer, Caroline, 1983, 'Pathan Women in Bradford: factors affecting mental health with reference to racism', in Burke, Aggrey (ed*), Transcultural Psychiatry: Racism and Mental Illness,* '30ᵗʰ Anniversary Double Issue of the International Journal of Social Psychiatry' Vol 30. 1-2, pp72-76.

— 2001, 'Is grief an illness? Issues of theory in relation to cultural diversity and the grieving process.' In Hockey, J, J Katz and N Small, pp49-60.

Culley, Lorraine, 1996, 'A critique of multiculturalism in health care: the challenge for nurse education', *The Journal of Advanced Nursing*, 1996, 23, 564-570.

Cutliffe, John R, 2000, 'Methodological issues in grounded theory', *Journal of Advanced Nursing,* 2000, 31(6), 1476-1484.

Dalley, Gillian, 2000, *Achieving a Good Death in London,* Centre for Policy on Ageing/Kings Fund.

Daly, Max, 1997, 'The throwaway grandmothers', *The Big Issue,* May 26-June 1, No 234.

Dean, Hartley, and Zafar Khan, 1998, 'Islam: A challenge to welfare professionalism', *Journal of Interprofessional Care*, Vol 12, No 4, 1998.

De Cock, Kevin M, Nicola Low, 1997, 'HIV and AIDS, other sexually transmitted diseases and tuberculosis in ethnic minorities in the United Kingdom: is surveillance serving its purpose?' *BMJ:* 314, 14 June, 1997, 1747-1751.

Del Amo, J, *et al.*, 1996, 'Spectrum of disease in Africans with AIDS in London', *Population Trends*, 1996, Summer (84) 33-39.

Dein, S, and J Stygall, 1997, 'Does being religious help or hinder coping with chronic illness? A critical literature review', *Palliative Medicine*, 291-298.

Dennis, Geoffrey, 1999 'Love is as strong as death: meeting the pastoral needs of the Jewish hospice patient', *American Journal of Hospice and Palliative Care,* 16(4) July/Aug, 1999:598-604.

Department of Health (DOH) 1992a, The *Health of the Nation,* London, HMSO

— 1992b, *The Patient's Charter*, London, HMSO

— 1998a, *Directory of African Caribbean Initiatives,* London, HMSO

— 1998b, *Directory of Asian Initiatives*, London, HMSO.

Dickenson, Donna, Malcolm Johnson and Jeanne Katz, pp183-191, *Death, Dying and Bereavement,* London, Open University and Sage Publications, 2001, 2ⁿᵈ edition.

Dom, Henry, 1999, 'Spiritual care, need and pain, recognition and response', *European Journal of Palliative Care*, 1999, 6(3): 87-90.

Douglas, Jenny, 'Developing appropriate research methodologies with black and ethnic minority communities, Part I: reflections on the research process', *Health Education Journal,* 1998 Dec 57(4): 329-38

Dowd, Steven B, V L Poole, K R Davidhizar and J N Giger, 1995, 'Dying, Death and Grief in a Transcultural context: application of the Giger and Davidhizar assessment model', *Hospice Journal,* Vol 13 (4) 33-46.

Doyle, Derek, Geoffrey W D Hanks, Neil MacDonald, (eds), 1998, *Oxford Textbook of Palliative Medicine,* 2nd Ed, Oxford University Press.

Easmon, Charles, 1999, 'Commentary: Isolate the problem, response to Selby', *BMJ,* 1999:318:1130

Ebrahim, Shah, 1996. 'Ethnic Elders', *BMJ,* Sept 7, 313, 705-76.

Eisenbruch, Maurice, 1984a, 'Cross-cultural Aspects of Bereavement I: A Conceptual Framework for Comparative Analysis', *Culture, Medicine and Psychiatry,* 8 (3) Sept:283-309.

— 1984b, 'Cross-Cultural, Aspects of Bereavement II: Ethnic and Cultural Variations in the Development of Bereavement Practices', *Culture, Medicine and Psychiatry,* 8 (4), Dec:315-347.

Elwin, Todd S, Michael D Fetters, Daniel W Gorenflo and Tsukasa Tsuda, 1998, 'Cancer disclosure in Japan: historical comparisons current practices' *Social Science and Medicine,* 46:115-116.

Ernst, Gernot, 2000, 'The myth of the "Mediterranean syndrome": do immigrants feel different pain?', *Ethnicity and Health,* 2000 5(2): 121-126

Erwin, Jo, and Barry Peters, 1999, 'Treatment issues for HIV in Africans in London,' *Social Science and Medicine,* 49, 1519-1528.

Eve, Ann, Anthony M Smith, Peter Tebbit, 1997, 'Hospice and palliative care in the UK 1994-1995, including a summary of trends 1990-1995', *Palliative Medicine,* 1997: 11:31-43.

Eve, Anne, and Irene J Higginson, 2000, 'Minimum dataset activity for hospice and hsopital palliative care services in the UK 1997/98', *Palliative Medicine,* 14: 395-404.

Fassil, Johannes, 1996 *'Primary Health Care for Black and Minority Ethnic People: a Consumer Perspective,'* NHS Ethnic Health Unit, 1996.

Fenton, Steve, 1999, *Ethnicity, Racism, Class and Culture,* Basingstoke, Macmillan.

Field, David, and Gina Copp, 1999, 'Communication and awareness about dying in the 1990s', *Palliative Medicine;* 13: 459-468.

Field, David, Jenny Hockey and Neil Small, 1997, *Death, Gender and Ethnicity,* London, Routledge

Field, D, and J Addington-Hall, 2000, 'Extending specialist palliative care to all?', *Social Science and Medicine,* 1999, Vol 48, pp1271-1280, reproduced in *Death and Dying: Offprints,* Open University, 2000.

Field, D and Chris Smaje, 1997, 'Absent minorities? Ethnicity and the use of palliative care services, in Field *et al.,* pp142-165.

Fielding, R, L Wong and L Ko, 1998, 'Strategies of information disclosure to Chinese cancer patients in an Asian community', *Psycho-social Oncology,* 7: 240-51

— 1999, Abstract in *Palliative Medicine,* 13:85-88

Firth, Shirley, 1993, 'Approaches to Death in Hindu and Sikh communities in Britain', in D Dickenson and M Johnson, (eds.) *Death, Dying and Bereavement,* London: Sage, pp26-32.

— 1997, *Dying, Death and Bereavement in a British Hindu Community*, Leuven, Peeters

— 1999a, 'Hindu widows in Britain: continuity and change', in Barot, Rohit, Steve Fenton and Harriet Bradley, (eds), pp99-114.

— 1999b, 'Spirituality and Ageing in British Hindus, Sikhs and Muslims' in Jewell, Albert, (ed), pp158-174.

— 2001, 'Hindu Death and Mourning Rituals: the impact of Geographic Mobility', in Hockey, J, and N Small (eds), pp237-246.

Flavin, C, 'Cross-cultural training for nurses,' *American Journal of Hospice and Palliative Care*, 14.3:121-6.

Foolchand, M K, 2000, 'The role of the Department of Health and other key institutions in the promotion of equal opportunities, multi-cultural and anti-racist issues in nurse education', *Nurse Education Today*, 2000, 20, 443-448.

Fountain, Averil, 1999, 'Ethnic minorities and palliative care in Derby', *Palliative Medicine* 1999: 13: 161-162.

Free, Caroline, 'Breaking down language barriers: some ethnic groups may have problems in getting as far as a consultation'. Letter in *BMJ* Sept 19, 1997, Vol 317. p816-7.

Froggatt, Katherine A, 2001, 'Palliative care and nursing homes', *Palliative Medicine*, 15:42-48.

Gaffin, J, D Hill and D Penso, 1996, 'Cancer and Ethnic minorities – the Department of Health's Perspective', *British Journal of Cancer* 74, Supp xxixx:551-553.

Gardner, Katy, 1998, 'Death, burial and bereavement amongst Bengali Muslims', *Journal of Ethnic and Migration Studies*, Vol 24, No 3, 507-521.

— 2001, *Age, Migration and Narrative: Bodies and the Life Course Amongst Bengali Elders in London*, Oxford, Berg, forthcoming.

Garner, M, 'Double Jeopardy: Asylum Seekers in Britain', *Community Care*, 6-12 Nov 1997, p25

Gerrish, Kate, 1997, 'Preparation of nurses to meet the needs of an ethnically diverse society: educational implications', *Palliative Medicine*, 17:359-365.

Gerrish, Kate, Charles Husband and Jennifer Mackenzie, 1996, *Nursing for a Multi-ethnic Society*, Buckingham, Open University Press.

Gerrish, Kate, 1999, 'Inequalities in service provision: an examination of institutional influences on the provision of district nursing care to minority ethnic communities', *Journal of Advanced Nursing*, Vol 30:6:1263-71, Dec 30.

Gibbs, L M E, J E Ellershaw and M D Williams, 1997, 'Caring for patients with HIV disease: the experience of a generic hospice', *Aids Care*, Vol 9, 5, 601-607.

Gill, Paramjit, Glen Scrivener, David Lloyd, and Tony Dowell, 1995, 'The effect of patient ethnicity on prescribing rates', *Health Trends*, Vol 27, 4, 111-113.

Gilliat-Ray, Sophie, 2000, 'Spirituality and the nursing profession', paper given at the 'Worship in Birmingham Project, "Spirituality" in Contemporary Britain', University of Birmingham, June 2000.

Gizer, J, and Davidhizar, R, 1995, *Transcultural Nursing: Assessment and Intervention*, St Louis, Mosby Year Book.

Glickman, M, 1997, *Making Palliative Care Better: Quality Improvement, Multi-professional Audit and Standards*, Occasional Paper 12, London, NCHSPS.

Gocoldas, Ila, 'Black and minority ethnic community access to hospice and palliative care services in Birmingham', abstract, personal communication by email.

Gordon, Deborah R, and Eugenio Paci, 1997, 'Disclosure Practices and Cultural narratives: understanding concealment and silence around cancer in Tuscany, Italy', *Social Science and Medicine*, 44:1433-1452.

Gorman, Audrey K, 'Hospice and minorities: a national study of organizational access and practice', *The Hospice Journal*, 11(1) 1996.

Gough, Pippa, 1999, 'Commentary: Courteous containment is not enough', response to Selby, *BMJ*, 1999:318:1131

Greater London Authority, 2000, *Without Prejudice? Exploring ethnic differences in London: Key Findings.*

Greenahalgh, Trisha, Cecil Helman, A Mu'min Chowdhury, 1998, 'Health beliefs and folk models of diabetes in British Bangladeshis; a qualitative study', *BMJ* March 1998, Vol 316, pp978-993.

Gunaratnam, Yasmin, 1997, 'Culture is not enough: a critique of multi-culturalism in palliative care', in Field, David, Jenny Hockey and Neil Small (eds), pp166-186.

1998, 'Re-thinking multicultural service provision, *Hospice Bulletin*, Aug 1998, 7-8

— 2001a, ' "We mustn't judge people... but": Staff dilemmas in dealing with racial harassment amongst hospice service users', *Sociology of Health and Illness* 2001: 23 (1), 65-83.

— 2001b, 'Ethnicity and Palliative Care', in L Culley and S Dyson, (eds), *Sociology, Ethnicity and Nursing Practice*, Palgrave, Forthcoming.

— 2001c, ' Working Across Cultures of Difference: Ethnicity and the Challenge for Palliative Day Care', in J Hearn and C Meyers (eds), *Palliative Day Care in Practice*, Oxford, Oxford University Press, Forthcoming.

— 2001d, 'Eating into multiculturalism: hospice staff and service users talk food, 'race' ethnicity, culture and identity', in *Critical Social Policy* 21(2) 253-276.

Gunaratnam, Yasmin, Isobel Bremner, Louis Pollock and Catherine Weir, 1998, 'Anti-discrimination, emotions and professional practice', *European Journal of Palliative Care,* 1998: 5(4).

Haffner 1992, 'Translation is not enough. Interpreting in a medical setting: Cross Cultural Medicine – a Decade Later', (special issue*) Western Journal of Medicine*, Sept 157, 255-259.

Hall, Pippa, Gail Stone, and Valerie J Fiset, 1998, 'Palliative Care: How can we meet the needs of our multicultural communities?' *Journal of Palliative Care* 14:2, 1998: 46-49.

Harding, S, 1998, 'The incidence of cancer among second generation Irish living in England and Wales: a longitudinal study', *British Journal of Cancer.* 78 (7):958-961.

Harding, S, and R Balarajan, 1996, 'Patterns of mortality in second generation Irish living in England and Wales: a longitudinal study', *BMJ*, 312:1389-1392.

Harding, S, and R Maxwell, 1997, 'Differences in the mortality of migrants' in Drever, F, and M Whitehead (eds), *Health Inequalities Decennial [Supplement]*, pp108-121, HMSO, London.

Harding, S. and Michael Rosato, 1999, 'Cancer Incidence among first generation Scottish, Irish, West Indian and South Asian Migrants Living in England and Wales', *Ethnicity and Health,* 1999, 491/2, 83-92.

Haringey Council, *Refugees and Asylum Seekers in Haringey: Research project report.* London: Haringey Council, 1997

Harper, Mary S, 1995, 'Caring for the special needs of ageing minorities', *Healthcare Trends and Transition*, Feb-Mar 1995, Vol 6, No 4.

Haskey, J, 1996, 'The ethnic minority populations of Great Britain; their estimated size and age profiles', *Population Trends*, Summer 1996, (84) 33-39.

Haworth, M, R Leonard, A Sadiq, 1997, 'Asian interpreters and palliative care', *Palliative Medicine,* 11:1:77.

Haworth, E A, V Soni Raleigh and R Balarajan, 1999, 'Cirrhosis and primary liver cancer among first generation migrants in England and Wales', *Ethnicity and Health*, 4 (1/2); 91-93.

Hawthorne, Kamila, 1994, 'Accessibility and use of health care Services in the British Asian Community', *Family Practice*, 11.4, 453-459.

Haroon-Iqbal, H, D Field, H Parker, and Z Iqbal, 1995, 'The absent minority: access and use of palliative care services by black and ethnic minority groups in Leicester', in A Richardson and J K Wilson-Barnett (eds), pp83-96.

Haskey, J, 1996, 'The Ethnic Minority Populations of Great Britain: their estimated size and age profiles', *Population Trends,* Summer (84) 33-9

Hayward, A, *Tuberculosis Control in London: The Need for change. A Report for the Thames Regional Directors of Public Health.* London: NHS Executive

Hearn, J, 1997, 'Trends in the place of death of cancer patients over 10 years: focus on patients born outside UK.' Unpublished MSc. Dissertation, University of London.

Heaven, Cathy and Peter Maguire, 1997, 'Disclosure of concerns by hospice patients and their identification by nurses', *Palliative Medicine*, 1997, 11: 283-290.

Helman, Cecil, 1994, *Culture, Health and Illness*, Oxford, Butterworth-Heinemann Ltd.

Henley, Alex, 1982, *Caring for Muslims and their Families*, London: DHSS/Kings Fund.

— 1983a, *Caring for Sikhs and their Families*, London: DHSS/Kings Fund.

— 1983b, *Caring for Hindus and their Families,* London: DHSS/Kings Fund.

— 1987, *Caring in a Multiracial Society*, London: DHSS/Kings Fund

Hern, H Eugene, Barbara A Koenig, Lisa Jean Moore and Patricia A Marshall, 1998, 'The difference that culture can make in end-of-life decision-making', *Cambridge Quarterly of Healthcare Ethics*, 7, 27-40.

Hill, Dawn, and Dawn Penso, 1995, *Opening Doors: Improving access to Hospice and Specialist Palliative Care Services by members of the Black and Ethnic Minority Communities,* National Council for Hospice and Specialist Palliative Care Services.

Hoare, Tanya, 'Breast cancer' in Rawaf, Salman and Veena Bahl, (eds), pp265-280

Hockey, Jenny, Jeanne Katz and Neil Small, 2001, *Grief, Mourning and Death Ritual*, Buckingham, Open University Press.

Hopwood, A L, 'The social construction of illness and its implications for complementary and alternative medicine', *Complementary Therapies in Medicine*, 1997, 5, 152-155.

Horn, S and M Musafo, 1997, *Pain: Theory, Research and Intervention*, Open University Press.

Hornberger, John *et al.*, 1996, 'Eliminating language barriers for non-English-speaking patients', *Medical Care*, Vol 34(8): 845-856.

Huang, X, P Butow, B Meiser, D Goldstein, 1999, 'Attitudes and information needs of Chinese migrant Cancer patients', *Austr.-N.Z Med*, April 29:2:207-13.

Irish, Donald P, Kathleen F Lundquist and Vivian Jenkins Nelson, (eds), *Ethnic Variations in Dying, Death and Grief, Diversity in Universality*, London, Taylor and Francis Ltd.

Islington Zairian Refugees Group. *Islington Zairian Refugees Survey Report.* London: Healthy Islington 2000

Jewell, Albert, (ed), 1999, *Ageing and Spirituality*, Jessica Kingsley.

Jeyasingham, Mercy, 2000, Health Advocacy, Presentation at NCHSPCS Symposium, Dec 2000.

Jones, David and Paramjit Gill, 1998, 'Breaking down barriers: The NHS needs to provide accessible interpreting services for all', *BMJ* May 16, Vol 316, p1476 (see Free's response).

Jonker, Gerdien, 1996, 'The knife's edge: Muslim burial in the diaspora', *Mortality* 1, I, 27-45.

— 1997, 'The many facets of Islam: death, dying and disposal between orthodox rule and historical convention', in Parkes, Colin Murray, Pittu Laungani and Bill Young, (eds) pp147-165).

Juarez, G, B Ferrell, and T Borneman, 1999, 'Cultural considerations in education for pain management', *Journal of Cancer Education*, 14(3): 168-73, Fall.

Kalsi, Sewa Singh, 1996, 'Change and continuity in the funeral rituals of Sikhs' in Howarth, Glennys and Peter C. Jupp, pp30-46.

Kanchandani R, and S Gillam, 1998, 'The Ethnic Minority Linkworker: a Key member of the Primary Health Care Team', cited Levinson and Gillam, 1998, in press.

Kai, Joe, 1999, 'Valuing ethnic diversity in primary care', *British Journal of General Practice*, Mar 1999.

Karim Kelvin, Maria Bailey and Kate Tunna, 1999, *Black/Minority Ethnic Communities and Hospice Care in Birmingham*, NHS Executive (W. Midlands), Primary and Community Care Research Initiative.

— 2000, 'Non-white ethnicity and the provision of specialist palliative care services: factors affecting doctors' referral patterns', *Palliative Medicine* 2000:14:471-478.

Karlson, Saffron, and Julia Addinton-Hall, 1998, 'How do cancer patients who die at home differ from those who die elsewhere?' *Palliative Medicine*, 12:279-286.

Karseras, P, and E Hopkins, 1987, *British Asians' Health in the Community*, Chichester: John Wiley.

Kashiwagi, Tetsuo, 'Palliative care in Japan', in Doyle *et al.* (eds), pp797-798

Katz, Jeanne Samson, 1996, 'Caring for dying Jewish people in a multicultural/ religious society', *International Journal of Palliative Nursing*, 1996, 2 (1).

— 2000, *Caring for Dying People,* Death and Dying (K260), Workbook 2, Open University, Buckingham, Open University Press.

— 2001, 'Jewish perspective on death, dying and bereavement', in Dickenson, Donna, Malcolm Johnson and Jeanne Katz, pp183-191

Kernohan, Elizabeth E M, 1998, 'Heart health', in Rawaf, Salman, and Veena Bahl (eds.), pp253-264.

Klass, D, 'The deceased child in the psychic and social worlds of bereaved parents during the resolution of grief', *Death Studies*, 21(2):147-75.

Kleinman A, 1977, 'Depression, somatisation and the new "cross-cultural psychiatry"', *Social Science and Medicine*, 11:3-10.

— 1986, *Social Origins of Distress and Disease: Neurasthenia and Pain in Modern China.* New Haven: Yale University Press.

King, Beattie, 1999, 'Caring for African clients with HIV', *Nursing Management*, Vol 6, No 6, Oct 1999

Kingsley, Su, nd. *Funding Initiative for Improving Health Among Ethnic Minority Populations,* Programme proposal.

Kite, Suzanne, Kate Jones, Adrian Tookman, 1999, 'Specialist palliative care and patients with noncancer diagnoses: the experience of a service' *Palliative Medicine*, 13:477-484.

Koffman, Jonathan, 1998, 'There must be a better way', *BMJ*. 316:1989-1990.

— 1999, Research: 'Care in the last year of life: comparing the experience of first generation black Caribbeans with the local white population in Lambeth', *Hospice Bulletin*, July 1999:3.

— 2000, 'Minority ethnic groups and *Our Healthier Nation', Journal of Public Health Medicine*, 22(2): 245-248.

Koffman, J, I Higginson and R Dunlop, Abstract: 'Care in the last year of life: satisfaction with health services among the Black Caribbean population in an inner London health authority', *Palliative Medicine*, 1999, 13:522.

Koffman, Jonathan and Irene Higginson, 2001, 'Accounts of satisfaction with health care at the end of life: a comparison of first generation black Caribbeans and white patients with advanced disease', accepted by *Palliative Medicine.*

Krause, I, 1989, 'The sinking heart, a Panjabi Communication of Distress', in *Social Science and Medicine,* 29 (4): 563-575.

Kübler-Ross, Elisabeth, 1970, *On Death and Dying,* London: Tavistock

— (ed) 1975, *Death: the Final Stage of Growth*, Englewood Cliffs, N J, Prentice Hall.

Laungani, Pittu, 1996, 'Death and Bereavement in India and England: a comparative analysis', *Mortality,* 1, (3): 191-211

— 1997, 'Death in a Hindu Family' in Parkes, Colin Murray, Pittu Laungani and Bill Young, (eds), pp52-71.

Leather, Chris and Sheila Wirz,1996, *The Training and Development Needs of Bilingual Support Workers in the NHS in Community Settings,* Centre for International Child Health, Institute of Child Health, London

Lees, S, and I Papadopoulos, 2000, 'Cancer and men from minority ethnic groups: an exploration of the literature', *European Journal of Cancer Care*, 9, 221-229.

Leininger, Madeleine, 1996, Response to Cooney Article, 'A Comparative Analysis of transcultural nursing and cultural safety.' *Nursing Praxis in New Zealand,* July 1996, 22 (2):13-15.

Levenson, R, and S Gillam, 1998, *Linkworkers in Primary Care,* London, King's Fund.

Levine, Ellen, 1997, 'Jewish views and customs on death', in Parkes, Colin Murray, Pittu Laungani and Bill Young, (eds), pp98-130.

Li, Piu-Ling, 1998, 'The Chinese experience' in Rawaf, Salman and Veena Bahl (eds), pp339-346.

Li, Piu-Ling , Stuart Logan, Lydia Yee and Sarah Ng, 1999, 'Barriers to meeting the mental health needs of the Chinese Community', *Journal of Public Health Medicine*, Vol 21, No 1.

Liao Xiao-hui and G McIlwaine, 1995, 'The health status and health needs of Chinese population in Glasgow', *Scottish Medical Journal* ,1995; 40:77-8.

Lindsay, James, Carol Jagger, Mark J Hibbert, Susan M Peet and Farida Moledina, 1997, 'Knowledge, uptake and availability of health and social services among Asian Gujarati and white elderly persons', *Ethnicity and Health*, 1997:2(1/2): 59-69

Lowdell, Caroline, Maria Evandrou, Martin Bardsley, David Morgan, Michael Soljak, *Health of Ethnic Minority Elders in London: Respecting Diversity*, July 2000. Health of Londoners Project.

Ludwig-Beymer, Patti 1998, 'Transcultural Aspects of Pain', in Andrews, Margaret M and Joyceen S Boyle (eds), pp283-307.

Lynam, J, 1992, 'Towards the goal of providing culturally sensitive care: principles upon which to build nursing curricula', *Journal of Transcultural Nursing*, 17, 149-57.

Madhok, Rajan, Aqueela Hameed and Raj Bhopal, 1998, 'Satisfaction with health services among the Pakistani population in Middlesborough, England', *Journal of Public Health Medicine*, Vol 20, No 3, pp295-301.

Mak, R, R Mwanje and A Pzniak, 1997, 'Issues facing Africans in London with HIV infection', Editorial, *Genitourinary Medicine*, 73: 157-158.

Marin, Isabelle, Nicole Dizengremel and Sylvie Fornasier, 1996, 'Returning foreign patients to their home country', *European Journal of Palliative Care*, 1996: 3(4):158-63.

Marmot, M G, Adelstein A M and Bulusu L, 1984, 'Immigrant Mortality in England and Wales 1970-1978', *Studies on Medical and Population Subjects* No 47, Office of Population Censuses and Surveys HMSO, London.

Mason, Dadid, 2000, *Race and Ethnicity in Modern Britain*, Oxford, Oxford University Press.

Melsack, Ronald, and Patrick D Wall. 'Pain mechanisms: a new theory'. Science 150, 971-979, 1965.

McCarthy, M, M. Lay and J Addington-Hall, 1996, 'Dying from Heart disease', *Journal of the Royal College of Physicians*, 30:325-328.

McCormick, A, D Fleming and J Charlton, 1995, *Morbidity Statistics from General Practice: Fourth National Study*, London: HMSO

McDonald, R, D Free, F Ross, and P Mitchell, 1998; 'Client preferences for HIV inpatient care delivery', *AIDS Care*, 10, supp 2, 1998, S123-S135.

McGarrigle, C A, and A Nicoll, 1998, 'Prevalence of HIV-1 among attenders at a sexually transmitted disease clinics: analysis according to country of birth', *Sex. Transm. Inf.* Dec 74 (6) 415-20.

McGrath, Pam, 1997, 'Spirituality and discourse: a postmodern approach to hospice research', *Australian Health Review*, 12:4:269-271.

— 1998, 'A spiritual response to the challenge of routinization: a dialogue of discourses in a Buddhist-initiated Hospice', *Qualitative Health Research*, 18(6), Nov:801-812.

McMunn, A, Roy Mwanje , Anton L Pzniak, 1997, 'Issues facing Africans in London with HIV infection' (editorial) *Genitourinary Medicine*, June, 73(3) 157-8.

McNamara, Beverley, Karen Martin, Charles Waddell, Kevin Yuen, 1997, 'Palliative care in a multicultural society: perceptions of health care professionals', *Palliative Medicine*, 1997, 359-367.

Melsack, Ronald, and Patrick D Wall, 1965, 'Pain mechanisms: a new theory', *Science*, 150:971-979.

Milne, Sheila Ann, 2000, 'The development and testing of a questionnaire to determine the understanding of and attitudes to palliative care services by the Chinese community'. Unpublished dissertation for MSc (Health Psychology), S'ton U.

Modood, Tariq, 1992, *Not Easy Being British*, Stoke on Trent, Trentham Books.

Modood, T, R Berthoud, J Lakey, J Nazroo, P Smith, S Vjirdee and S Beishon, 1997, *Ethnic Minorities in Britain,* London, Policy Studies Institute.

Moore, Rodney A, and Samuel F Dworkin, 1988, 'Ethnographic methodologic assessment of pain perceptions by verbal descriptions', *Pain* 1988, 195-204.

Mount, John, 2000, Proposal for research: To investigate the palliative care needs of ethnic minority groups in the local community, St. Catherine's Hospice, Crawley.

Mugisha, Richard and Sarah Nansukusa, 1998. 'The African Experience', in Rawaf, Salman and Veena Bahl (eds) pp329-338.

Murphy, Kathy and Jill Macleod Clark, 1993, 'Nurses experiences of caring for ethnic minority clients', *Journal of Advanced Nursing*, 18, 442-450.

Narayanasamy, Aru, 1999a, 'Transcultural mental health nursing 1: benefits and limitations', *British Journal of Nursing*, 8(10), 664-668.

— 1999b, 'Transcultural mental health nursing 2: Race, ethnicity and culture', *British Journal of Nursing*, 8(11), 741-744.

Nazroo, James Y, 1997a, *'Ethnicity and Mental health: Findings from a National Community Survey',* Policy Studies Institute.

— 1997b, *The Health of Britain's Ethnic Minorities,* London, Policy Studies Institute

Neuberger, Julia, 1998, 'Introduction', in Doyle *et al.* (eds), pp777-785.

— 1999a, 'Judaism and palliative care', *European Journal of Palliative Care*, 1999, 6(5).

— 999b, *Dying Well: a Guide to Enabling a Good Death*, Hale, Hochland & Hochland.

— 1999c, 'Commentary: a role for personal values… and management' a response to Selby, *BMJ,* 1999:318:1130.

Ng, N F, Anne Shumacker and G B Goh, 2000, 'Autonomy for whom? A perspective from the Orient', *Palliative Medicine* 14:163-164.

NHS Ethnic Health Unit, 1996a, *Good Practice and Quality Indicators in Primary Health Care: Health Care for Black and Minority Ethnic People,*

Noggle, Barbara, 1995, 'Identifying and Meeting Needs of Ethnic Minority Patients', *Hospice Care and Cultural Diversity,* 10 (2),85-93.

Notta, Hardev and Brian Warr, 1998, 'Acorns Children's Hospice, Birmingham' in Oliviere *et al.*, pp148-150.

Nwoga, I A, 1994, 'Traditional healers and perceptions of the causes and treatment of cancer'. *Cancer Nursing*, 17, 470-478.

Nursing Standard Report, 1998, 'Nursing older people from ethnic minority communities,' Vol 12, No 51, pp29-30.

Office of Population Censuses and Surveys, Census 91 CM 17/1, 1991, Inner London, HMSO.

Ohara, Shin, 2000, 'We-consciousness and terminal patients: some biomedical reflections on Japanese civil religion', in Becker, Gerhold K (ed), *The Moral Status of Persons: Perspectives on Bioethics,* Amsterdam – Atlanta Ga., Rodopi.

Ohynuki-Tierney, E, 1984, *Illness and Culture in Contemporary Japan: An Anthropological View,* Cambridge, Cambridge University Press.

Oliviere, David, 1999 'Culture and ethnicity', *European Journal of Palliative Care,* 6(2), 53-56.

Oliviere, David, Rosalind Hargreaves and Barbara Monroe, 1998, *Good Practices in Palliative Care: a Psychosocial Perspective,* Aldershot, Ashgate Arena.

Olweny, Charles L M, 1998, 'Cultural issues in sub-Saharan Africa', in Doyle *et al.*, 787-791.

Papadopoulos, Irena, 1998, 'The health needs of Greek Cypriot People', in Papadopoulos, Irena, Mary Tilki and Gina Taylor, pp80-162.

Papadopoulos, Irena, Mary Tilki and Gina Taylor, 1998, *Transcultural Care: a Guide for Health Care Professionals,* Salisbury, Quay Books.

Papadopoulos, Irena and Jo Alleyne, 1998, 'Health of minority ethnic groups', in Papadopoulos, Irena, Mary Tilki and Gina Taylor, pp1-17.

Papadopoulos, Irena, Mary Tilki and Gina Taylor, 'Developing transcultural skills' in Papadopoulos, Irena, Mary Tilki and Gina Taylor, pp186-222

Parekh *et al.*, 2000, *The Future of Multi-Ethnic Britain,* report of the Commission on the Future of Multi-Ethnic Britain, the Runnymede Trust, London, Profile Books.

Parkes, Colin Murray, 1972, *Bereavement: Studies of Grief in Adult Life,* London, Tavistock.

Parkes, Colin Murray, Pittu Laungani and Bill Young, (eds), 1997, *Death and Bereavement Across Cultures ,* London, Routledge.

Patel, Naina, 1999, 'Black and minority elderly perspectives on long-term care', in, *Royal Commission on Long-term Care, With Respect to Old Age: Long term Care- Rights and Responsibilities,* London, the Stationary Office.

Pfeffer, N, and K C Moynihan, 'Ethnicity and health beliefs with respect to cancer: a critical review of methodology,' *British Journal of Cancer,* 1996, 74, supp XXIX, S66-S72.

Pharoah, K, 1995, *Primary Health Care for Elderly People from Black and Minority Ethnic Communities,* HMSO.

Phelan, M and S Parkinson, 1995, 'How to work with an interpreter', *BMJ,* 311:555-557.

Pilgrim, S, S Fenton, T Hughes, C Hine and N Tibbs, 1993, *The Black and Ethnic Minorities Health Survey Report,* Bristol, University of Bristol.

Pincombe, J, M Brown, D Thorne, A. Ballantyne and H McCutcheon, 2000, 'Care of dying patients in the acute hospital', *Progress in Palliative Care* 8(2) 2000

Pitches, David, 2000, *Health Services in Birmingham for Black and Minority Ethnic Older People: Report of a Baseline Survey for Birmingham Race Action Partnership,* Aug 2000, Birmingham Health Authority.

Polaschek, N R, 1998, 'Cultural safety: a new concept in nursing people of different ethnicities', *Journal of Advanced Nursing,* 1998, 27, 452-457.

Pointon, Tom, 1996, 'Telephone interpreting service is available', *BMJ,* 1996, Jan 6, 312:53. Letter, response to Phelan and Parkman, *BMJ* 1995,3 22:555-7, Aug 26

Powell, J E, E Mendez, S E Parkes and J R Mann, 2000, 'Factors affecting survival in white/Asian children with leukaemia', *British Journal of Cancer*, 82; 3, 1568-70.

Prior, Deborah, 1999, 'Palliative Care in Marginalised Communities', *Progress in Palliative Care* 7(3):109-115.

Ramsden, I, 1990, *Kawawhakaruruhau: Cultural Safety in New Zealand*, Ministry of Education, Wellington.

— 1993, 'Kawawhakaruruhau, cultural safety in nursing education in Aorearoa (NZ), *Nursing Praxis*, 8(3) 4-10.

Raschid A, and C Jagger, 1992, 'Atitudes to a perceived use of health care services among Asian and non-Asian patients in Leicester', *British Journal of General Practice,* 42:197-120.

Rawaf, S, 1996, 'Assessing the health needs for cancer services for people from ethnic groups', *British Journal of Cancer* (1996) 74, Supp XXIX, S35-S37.

Rawaf, Salman and Veena Bahl (eds), 1998, *Assessing Health Needs of People from Minority Ethnic Groups,* Royal College of Physicians.

Rees, 1971, 'The hallucinations of widowhood', *BMJ*, 4:37-41.

— 1986, 'Immigrants and the hospice' *Health Trends*, 78:23-91.

— 1997, *Death and Bereavement: The Psychological, Religious and Cultural Interfaces*, London: Whurr.

Ritch, A E S, M Kehtisham, S Guthrie, J M Talbot, M Luckkl, R N Tinsley, 1996, 'Ethnic Influence on health and dependency of elderly inner city residents', 1996, *Journal of the Royal College of Physicians of London*, 30 (3), May/June:215-220.

Richardson, A, and J K Wilson-Barnett (eds), *Research in Cancer Nursing*, London: Scutari.

Rosenblatt, P C, 1993, 'Cross-cultural variations in the experience, expression and understanding of grief,* in Irish *et al.,* (eds.), pp13-20.

— 1997, 'Grief in small-scale societies', in Parkes, C M, P Laungani and B Young, (eds), pp27-51.

Rosenblatt, P C, R Walsh and D Jackson, 1976, *Grief and Mourning in Cross-cultural Perspectives,* Washington DC, HRAF Press.

Royal College of Nursing, 1998, *The Nursing Care of Older Patients from Black and Minority Ethnic Communities: a Royal College of Nursing Resource Guide.*

Rudack, K, 1994, 'Minority ethnic Groups in England. London': Health Education Authority (Health and Lifestyles).

Rudd, Anthony, F C Martin, A H Hopper, E Redmond and C Record, 1997, 'Community health care for South Asian elders', *Health Visitor*, Vol 70 (5): 182-184).

Sadler, Catherine, 1999, 'Promoting Diversity', *Nursing Standard,* June 16, 13 (39): 14-16.

Salt, S, L Wilson, and A Edwards, 1998, 'The use of specialist palliative care services by patients with human immunodeficiency virus-related illness in the Yorkshire Deanery of the Northern and Yorkshire region', *Palliative Medicine*:12:152-160.

Sahlberg-Blom, E, B-M Ternestedt, J-E Johansson, 1998, 'The last month of life: continuity, care site and place of death', *Palliative Medicine* 1998:12:287-296:

Schriever, Silvia H, 'Comparison of beliefs and practices of ethnic Viet and Lao Hmong concerning illness, healing, death and mourning: implications for hospice care with refugees in Canada', 1990, *Journal of Palliative Care* 6(1) 42-49.

Seale, Clive, 1998, *Constructing Death: the Sociology of Death and Bereavement*, Cambridge, Cambridge University Press.

Secretary of State for Health, 1999, *'Saving lives: our healthier nation'*, Cm 4386, London: the Stationery Office.

Selby, Mary, 1999, 'Ethical Dilemma: Dealing with racist patients', *BMJ*, 318:1129.

Sensky, T, 1996, 'Eliciting lay beliefs across cultures: principles and methodology'. *British Journal of Cancer*, 74, suppl XXIX, S63-S65.

Shah, Leena, Ian Harvey and Edward Coyle, 1998, 'Qualitative before quantitative' in Rawaf, Salman, and Veena Bahl (eds), pp35-55.

Shamash, Jack, 1998, 'Haunted Memories'. *Nursing Standard* March 18, 112 (26):26-27.

Shanahan, Mary, and D Lynett Brayshore, 1995, 'Are nurses aware of the differing health care needs of Vietnamese patients?' *Journal of Advanced Nursing*, 1995, 22, 456-464.

Shapiro, E, 1996, 'Family bereavement and cultural diversity: a social developmental model', *Family Process*, 35 (4):312-32.

Sharma, Kiran, 2000, 'A question of faith for the Hindu patient', *European Journal of Palliative Care*, 7(3) 99-100.

Shaw, Alison, 1999, *'Kinship and Continuity: Pakistani Families in Britain'*, Harwood Academic Press.

Sibley, Dennis, 1997, 'Caring for Dying Buddhists', *International Journal of Palliative Nursing*, Jan/Feb 1997 3(1):26-30

Siddell, M, J Katz and C Komaromy, 2000, *Death and Dying in Residential and Nursing Homes for Older People*, School of Health and Social Welfare, Open University, Buckingham.

Silvera, Mike and Rukshana Kapasi, *Health Advocacy for Minority Ethnic Londoners: Putting Services on the map?* 2000, London, Kings Fund/NHS Executive.

Sliviera, E R, S K Ebrahim, 1998, 'Social determinants of psychological morbidity and well-being in immigrant elders and whites in East London', *International Journal of Geriatric Psychiatry*, Nov, 133(11) :801-2

Simmonds, Rosemary, 2001, 'Improving access to Palliative Care Services for Ethnic Minority Groups', Progress Report for Research Group meeting, Wednesday 19 Jan, 2001.

Simmonds, Rosemary and John Mount, 2001, 'Minority ethnic groups are under-represented in palliative care… St. Catherine's Hospice in West Sussex asks 'Why' and 'What can we do to help?' Draft for *Information Exchange – Research and Education*.

Smaje, Chris, 1995, *Health, Race and Ethnicity, Making Sense of the Evidence*, Kings Fund Institute/Share.

Smaje, Chris and David Field, 1997, 'Absent minorities? Ethnicity and the use of palliative care services' in Field, David, J Hockey and N Small, pp142-165.

Smaje, Chris and Julian Le Grand, 'Ethnicity, equity and the use of health services in the British NHS', *Social Science and Medicine*, 45:3:485-496.

Small, Neil, *'Spirituality and Hospice Care'*, 1998, in Cobb, Mark, and Vanessa Robshaw (eds), pp. 167-182.

Smettem, Saram 'Welcome/Assalaam-u-alaikaam: 'Improving communications with ethnic minority families', *Paediatric Nursing* 11(2): Mar 1999:33-35.

Smith, Marcia Bayne, 1999, 'Primary Care: Choices and Opportunities for Racial/Ethnic Minority Populations in the USA and UK – a comparative analysis', *Ethnicity and Health* 1999: 4(3): 165-188.

Smith, J W, 1996, 'Cultural and religious Issues in palliative care', *Journal of Cancer Care,* Oct, 5(4); 173-8.

Sogyal Rimpoche, 1992, *The Tibetan Book of Living and Dying*, P Gaffney and A Harvey, (eds), San Francisco, Harper.

Somerville, J E, 2001, 'The Experience of Informal Carers Within the Bangladeshi Community', *Palliative Medicine,* 7 (5): 240-247..

Spruyt, Odette, 1999, 'Community-based palliative care for Bangladeshi patients in East London: Accounts of bereaved carers', *Palliative Medicine*, 1999, 13: 119-129.

Stansworth, Rachel, 1997, 'Spirituality, language and depth of reality', *International Journal of Palliative Nursing,* (3(1):19-22.

Staniszewska, S, L Ahmed, and C Jenkinson, 1999, 'The conceptual validity and appropriateness of using health-related quality of life measures in minority ethnic groups', *Ethnicity and Health,* 1999, 41/2 51-63.

Stephen, H, 1998, 'Shining through', *Nursing Standard,* Sept 30(13):14-15.

Still Building Bridges: the report of the national inspection of arrangements for the integration of care programme approach with care management, DOH/SSI 1999

Stroebe, M, and H Schut, 1998, 'Culture and Grief', *Bereavement Care*, 17(1): 7-11.

Specialist Palliative Care: 1995, *A Statement of Definitions*, Occasional Paper 8, London, National Council for Hospice and Specialist Palliative Care Services.

Swan, Elaine, 1999, 'Equal care for all', *Nursing Standard,* March 24, Vol 13, No 27:42-44.

Swerdlow, A J, M G Marmot, A K E Grulich and J Head, 1995, 'Cancer mortality in Indian and British ethnic immigrants from the Indian subcontinent to England and Wales', *British Journal of Cancer* 72:1312-1319.

Sze, Frank Kai-hoi, TK Chung, Eric Wong, KK Lam, Raymond Lo and Jean Woo, 1998, 'Pain in Chinese cancer patients under palliative care', *Palliative Medicine,* 1998, 12: 12: 271-277.

Tate, Colleen Wedderburn, 1996, 'All talk and no action', *Nursing Management,* Sept, 3 (5):7

Taylor, Andrew and Margaret Box, 1999, *Multicultural Palliative Care Guidelines,* Palliative Care Council of South Australia, 202 Greenhill Road, Eastwood, S. Australia 5063.

Taylor, Gina. *'Health and citizenship'*, 1998, in Papadopoulos, Irena, Mary Tilki and Gina Taylor, pp18-54

Tebbit, Peter. *'Palliative Care 2000 Commissioning Through Partnership',* London, NCHSPCS.

Tate, Coleen Wedderburn, 1996, 'All talk and no action,' *Nursing Management*, 3(5), Sept.

The Stephen Lawrence Inquiry and Home Secretary's Action Plan: Initial Guidance for Local Authorities, June 1999, Local Government Association,

They Look After Their Own, Don't They?: the report of the national inspection of community care services for black and ethnic minority older people, 1998, DOH/SSI.

Thomas, Veronica Nicky, 1997, 'Cancer and minority ethnic groups: factors likely to improve nurse-patient communication', *Journal of Cancer Nursing,* 1(3): 124-140.

Thompson, Katharine, 1998, 'Letter from Hong Kong', *Progress in Palliative Care',* 6(4) 116-117.

Thornhill Lee, Siew-Peng, 1999, 'Managing 'Face'; Hygiene and convenience at a Funeral in Singapore', Paper given at the conference, The Social Context of Death, Dying and Disposal, London University, 2000.

Tierney, Ryan M, Samuel M Horton, Terry J Hannan and William M Tierney, 1998:12:333-344. 'Relationships between symptom relief, quality of life and satisfaction with hospice care', *Palliative Medicine*, 1998, 12:333-344.

Tilki, Mary, 1998a, 'Old Age in Afro-Caribbean and Asian communities in Britain', in Papadopoulos, Irena, Mary Tilki and Gina Taylor, pp55-79.

— 1998b, 'The health of the Irish in Britain', in Papadopoulos, Irena, Mary Tilki and Gina Taylor, pp136-162.

Trevino, Fernando M, 'Quality of health care for ethnic/racial minority populations', 1999, *Ethnicity and Health* 1999, 4(3): 153-164.

Trive, Rachel, 1999, 'Bridging the gap or damming the flow? Some observations on using intepreters/bi-cultural workers when working with refugee clients, many of whom have been tortured', *British Journal of Medical Psychiatry,* 72: 567-576.

Twinn, Sheila, 1997, 'An exploratory study examining the influence of translation on the validity and reliability of qualitative data in nursing research', *Journal of* Advanced *Nursing,* 1997, 26, 418-423.

Vydelingum, Vasso, 1998, "'We treat them all the same' the experiences of nursing staff and of South Asian patients in a general hospital'*,* unpublished PhD, U. of Southampton.

— 2000, 'South Asian patients' lived experience of acute care in an English hospital: a phenomenological study', *Journal of Advanced Nursing,* 2000, 32(1) 100-107.

Walker, Caroline, 'Attitudes to death and bereavement among cultural minority groups', *Nursing Times,* Dec 15, 1982/

Walter, Tony, 1996, 'A new model of grief: bereavement and biography', Mortality, 1(1): 7-25.

— 1997, Developments in the spiritual care of the dying', *Religion*, 26;1-11.

— 1999, *On Bereavement*, Buckingham, Open University Press.

Warnakulasurya, K, N W Johnson, K Linklater and J Bell, 1999, 'Cancer of the mouth, pharynx and nasopharynx in Asian and Chinese immigrants resident in the Thames Region', published in *Oral Oncology* 35(5): 471-5, 1999, Sept.

Webb, Lalitha and Erica Young, 2000a, *Opening Doors to Better Palliative Care Services for People From a Culturally Diverse Community:* (Official): No exclusion clause project to improve access to palliative care services for people from a culturally diverse community (Warwickshire study).

— 2000b, *Opening Doors to Better Palliative Care Services for People from a Culturally Diverse Community*, NCHSPCS Symposium, London.

Webb, E, 1996, '*Meeting the needs of minority ethnic communities',* Archives of Disease in Childhood, 1996, Mar, 74(3) 264-7.

Weinstein, 1998: '*Community based counselling for the bereaved: a user based project'.* Alternative Health International, 1(2) Oct 1998. 3-16.

West Sussex Health Authority, *Pointers to Progress: Improving Health and Social Care for the People from Minority Ethnic Groups in the Crawley area,* Oct 1997.

White, C, 'Will the Glass Ceiling Shatter? A Worrying Trend Within Social Services – a Decrease in the Number of Black Senior Managers', *Community Care.* 17-23 Sept 1998, pp18-19

White D, K Phillips and A Minns, 1999, *Women from Ethnic Minority Communities: Their Knowledge of and Needs for Health Advocacy Services in East London.* Stoke-on-Trent: Staffordshire University Press, 1999

Wild, Sarah, Paul McKeigue, 197, 'Cross section analysis of mortality by country of birth in England and Wales', 1970-92, *BMJ,* 1997, Mar 8, Vol 314:705-713.

Wilkie, Patricia, 1997, 'Ethical issues in qualitative research in palliative care' *Palliative Medicine* 11, 321-324.

Wilkinson, E K, C Salisbury, N Bosanquet, P J Franks, S Kite, M Lorentzon, A Naysmith, 1999, 'Patient and carer preference for, and satisfaction with, specialist models of palliative care: a systematic literature review', *Palliative Medicine,* 199: 13: 197-216.

Winter, H, K K Cheng, C Cummins, R Maric, P Silcocks, and C Varghese, 1999, 'Cancer incidence in the South Asian population of England (1990-92)', *British Journal of Cancer,* 79 (3/4) 645-654).

Woo, K Y, 1999, 'Care for Chinese Palliative Patients', *Journal of Palliative Care,* 1999, 15(4): 70-4.

Worden, J W, 1991, *Grief counselling and Grief Therapy,* 2nd edn, London, Routledge/New York, Springer.

Wright, Bob, 'In favour of tolerance', Editorial, *Accidental and Emergency Nursing,* 1999, 7:129.

Wrightson, K J, and J Wardle, 1997, 'Cultural variation in health locus of control', *Ethnicity and Health,* 2(12):13-20.

Xueqin Ma, Grace, 1999, 'Between two worlds: the use of traditional and western health services by Chinese immigrants', *Journal of Community Health,* 24 (6), 421-437.

Yee, Lydia, 1997, '*Breaking Barriers Towards Culturally Competent General Practice: A consultation project for the GCGP Inner City Task Force*'. London, The Royal College of General Practitioners.

Zborowski, M,1952, 'Cultural components in response to pain', *Journal of Social Issues,* 8(16-30).

Zola, I K, 1966, 'Culture and symptoms: an analysis of patients' presenting complaints,' American Sociological Review. 31:615-630.

— 1966, 'Culture and symptom: an analysis of patients' presenting complaints', *American Sociological Review,* 31:615-630.